WE ARE
NOT
THE SAME

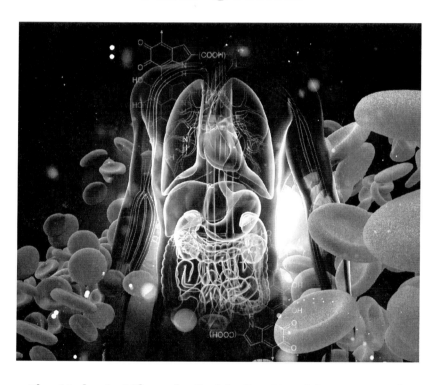

*The Melanin Lifestyle Guide For Nutrition, Mental,
And Spiritual Well-Being*

Shaneequewa Samuels

Instagram: Neequa_09

ISBN 978-1-54397-167-5 (print)
ISBN 978-1-54397-168-2 (eBook)

Note to Reader: The material presented here is for educational use only and should not be used as a substitute for professional medical advice, diagnosis, or treatment. Neither this nor any book should be used as substitute for professional care or treatment. The opinions and conclusions expressed in this book are mine, and unless expressed otherwise, mine alone. It is advisable to seek the guidance of a physician or other qualified health practitioner before implementing any of the approaches to health suggested in this book.

This book was written to provide selected information to the public concerning conventional and alternative medical treatments. Be advised that every person is unique and may respond differently to the treatments described in this book. On occasion I have provided dosage recommendations where appropriate. Neither the author, publisher, nor producer take any responsibility for any possible consequences from any treatment, action, or application of herbal treatment by any person reading or following information in this book.

My writings are to help guide you to live a healthy lifestyle and prevent health problems. If you suspect you have a medical problem, please seek alternative health professionals to help you make the healthiest, informed choices.

DEDICATION

To my amazing mother, **Shirley,** who raised me, my sister Samantha, and my brother Safaree all on her own. My inspiration to live a holistic natural lifestyle has been inspired by her from birth. Thank you for your knowledge and your greatness!

To my beautiful sister, **Samantha,** my brother **Devon**, and my amazing nieces, **Natanya** and **Naomi**. Samantha is one of the most beautiful and intelligent people I know and I always admired that about her.

My other half, **Safaree,** who is a true inspiration. There are not too many people I know that could have endured some of the things he has and still come out on top. Thank you for continuing to be a true inspiration and showing me not to stress over anything.

My daughter, **Melia**. Sometimes, I still can't believe I was part of your creation. You are a true miracle. Your happiness, your energy, and your lovingkindness at such a young age are something to be revered. I know you will grow up to be a strong, intelligent, and conscious Queen. My cousin, **Sophia**, is a true sweetheart. I was plotting to have you kidnapped when I was younger, but I truly love you and you have a big beautiful heart to go with that long belly of yours. I love you Cuzzo! Huge thanks to my other mother, **Mary "Ms. C" Aaron**, who takes care of my family and Melia as if she is her own. You have such a huge heart and I thank God that I met you!

Thank you to my entire family and all of my friends. Thank you to the readers who are ready to take a journey that will forever change their lives. My ancestors and the creator of all things, none of this could have been done without you. Thank you for aligning the universe for me to see my purpose. I LOVE YOU!

IN LOVING MEMORY OF
VINCENT "UNCLE VERN" ROPER

CONTENTS

INTRODUCTION

Over the years, you've probably put things in your body that are leaving a residue in your system, and are having a negative effect on your quality of life. You are allowing people who either don't know anything about you, or don't care enough to create a health system to benefit you to guide your health. Ladies and gentlemen, that's where I come in. I eat, breathe, and sleep the forward movement of people of color. You have been experimented on and neglected for centuries. America has some of the best medical and scientific advancements of the entire world, but still have the sickest population. Why?

The present work is a result of ten years of research and experimenting; and I'm not stopping here. I've done a lot of trial and error to figure out the perfect cleansing process/diet for family, friends, referred people, and myself. In the first section of this book, I'm going to lay out a step-by-step process of four ways to fully cleanse your body before changing your diet. Good health requires commitment, investment, and maintenance. You can't buy good health no matter how rich you are, the amount of degrees earned, or cars you have.

I'm not one to use too much fancy scientific terminology because I want to keep it as simple as possible. There will be some science, so please bear with me if this is all new to you. The medical industry wants to confuse you with their fancy words and jargon so you won't question their methods, but I assure you; it's much simpler than you think. Most diseases are lifestyle disease and a cure would take profits from one of the biggest industries in America – the multi-billion dollar medical/ pharmaceutical industry.

The first section of this book is all about melanin, nutrition, and cleansing. I address melanin because it's a critical reason why our communities aren't functioning at optimal levels. In a doctor's office, you can't prescribe the same course of treatment to someone of African/ Hispanic descent as you would to someone of European descent. You will soon learn that our bodies are not only different on the outside, but they are drastically different on the inside, down to the blood content. There's a great misunderstanding about the original diet of our ancestors. That will be cleared up for you in this work because it's very important to understand the best diet for an African person to function at peak levels.

The reason you cleanse first is so your body can absorb the nutrients from the nutritious food you're about to put in there. Without cleansing, it gets mixed in with the filth sitting in your digestive tract and doesn't get absorbed properly. Colon issues play an important role in health problems. It is the final filtration process your digestive system sends food through.

According to our medical community, it's normal to have a bowel movement anywhere from three times a day to three times a week. Three times a week! Absolutely not, because the food that is not being eliminated is sitting in your digestive tract rotting and turning into toxic waste. Typical foods like pizza, pasta, steak, and white rice have zero fiber, therefore slowing down the transition of the food from your mouth to your butt. Then you start having constipation, indigestion, and other intestinal tract issues. Once your body begins to get clogged up, your other organs will start to be affected and dis-ease will be introduced into your body.

Over-eating, putting food on top of food, processed food, late night eating, and snacking between meals are your first-class ticket to accelerated aging and dis-ease. These habits are destroying our melanin that needs specific nourishment. I don't believe in fad diets or radical approaches because they're not long lasting and typically aren't designed for melanin dominant individuals. What I want to introduce here is for a lifetime. I know a lot of people want the doctor to give them a magic pill to make all their aches and pains go away, but it isn't that simple. A doctor's sole function is to keep you comfortable in your disease so you can continuously patronize the pharmaceutical industry.

In the second section of this book, you will learn about the primary reason for debilitating health amongst people of color in America. The reason dates back over 400 years ago to when our ancestors were removed from their continent and brought to North America, South America, and the Caribbean for slave labor.

The slave trade is the sole reason for our terrible eating practices. Some of you may think just because you come from Trinidad, Jamaica, Haiti, DR, PR etc. that you're following the diets of your ancestors, but you're not. You're following a slave diet. My purpose in the second section is to break down our history before, during, and after slavery. This information will allow you to see the generational habits that need to be broken in order for you to have good spiritual, mental, and physical health. You're allowing people who don't know anything about you to educate you on your history. Mental ingestion of bad information is equally or more detrimental than physical ingestion of poor foods.

In the final section of this book, mental health will be addressed. This topic is constantly overlooked, but needed most in our community. The information in this section will allow you to slow down your thoughts to allow for self-control, assisting you in finding purpose in your life.

You will see some things in this book that are repetitive. I did that on purpose because I really want you to understand the information presented before you. Don't wait any longer. The sooner you make the changes in this book to become a self-healer, the faster you reverse the aging process and improve your overall health.

PART I:
REVERSING 400+ YEARS
OF DETERIORATING HEALTH

1

"THE BLACKER THE BERRY THE SWEETER THE JUICE"

People of color suffer worse health issues than any other race in America. We have the lowest life expectancy and the highest death rate of any racial group, due to the lack of concern or awareness about your bodies and health. There are several reasons for debilitating health amongst African American and Hispanic people with a few being: racial discrimination, lack of affordable health services, poor health education, and limited access to health insurance. We are the most physically, spiritually and mentally strong of any race, but are continuously getting knocked out of the race towards good health because of bad choices.

If the system of America was never made to have us on the other side of the finish line, it's time to create your own system and stop waiting for things to get better. A large majority of medical schools do not have a requirement to take even a single course on nutrition and the ones that do typically offer a 1 day course. You only get one body and you have to stay in it for the rest of your life, so let's take the necessary steps to prevent or reverse some of the leading causes of disease and death in America.

Heart disease is number one and cancer is number two. These are two things you have a great amount of control over. While medical science continues to treat the symptoms and not the cause, I want to help you treat the cause so we don't have to depend solely on our doctors. Western science has added great advancement towards medicine but it is still highly flawed. In acute situations, prescription drugs and surgery may have lifesaving capabilities. But over time it is imperative to transition to a holistic lifestyle. Sickness is a multi-billion dollar industry, so if you think a cure for anything is coming from some place outside of yourself, it's time to wake-up.

My purpose in this section is to show you how important it is to nourish what makes your skin brown to black, then give you several solutions to start taking steps towards great health. You are Gods on earth living and eating like slaves during the 1600's. These are not the original diets/foods of our ancestors. These were the scraps of our slave masters that you continue, by choice now, to put in your mouths. It's time to reverse the damage before America takes you out of the picture with their genetically modified foods, prescription drugs, processed foods, fast foods, and liquor stores that are flourishing all over our neighborhoods. The blacker the berry the sweeter the juice, but the way that an astounding number of men and women of color eat/drink, the berry is slowly rotting. This berry is called melanin and it's time for you to understand how important it is for getting you "right" mentally, physically, and spiritually.

WHAT IS MELANIN?

Many Greek philosophers who went to ancient Africa to study after the pyramids were built believed melanin played a major role in the intellect of African people. The reason our ancestors were able to construct those pyramids are because for millions of years, they studied nature and what diet was most suitable for our bodies that have the highest melanin content. They knew certain foods would alter our ability to achieve our highest level of performance.

We have been experimented on, studied, and murdered because they know more than you know that your melanin makes you powerful beyond measure. So why would they tell you anything about melanin? Instead they flood our neighborhoods with fast-food, Chinese restaurants, "chicken spots," liquor stores, and bodegas. Foods available in the black and brown communities are almost engineered to cause cancer, diabetes, heart disease, stroke and high blood pressure.

Medical science tells us that melanin is just a pigment that makes our skin, hair, and eyes brown or black. Fortunately, our African doctors and chemists have shown us that's not all it is. Dr. Llaila O. Afrika says "It is the chemical key to life."[1]

Melanin is a biochemical (living) substance found in all human beings internally and externally. Melanin is pigmented molecules that you can find in the atmosphere, the outer part of the earth, and in the universe, which leads to the ancient Egyptian proverb, "As above so below." This dark substance controls your emotional, physical, spiritual, and mental behavior.

"Germany, Italy, France, Japan and the US have a meeting about melanin every three to five years to discuss the latest research in melanin. They never invited a black scientist to that meeting."[2] I find it very interesting that no black scientists or melanin dominant countries are invited to a meeting where they are trying to learn about the main element in people of color. Or is it that they know how important melanin is, and how it affects us; but don't want the information distributed worldwide?

I want to use this entire section to summarize documentaries on melanin by some amazing black scientists and doctors; the keys to life that make us a "hue-man." This is information provided by Dr. Llaila O. Afrika, Dr. Jewel Pookrum, and Dr. Ann Brown. They have provided us with vital information that can bring great awareness to our race.

- Melanin is produced directly from the brain and cells known as melanocytes.

- Melanin causes brown and black children to have the fastest growth and development of any race... IF YOU NOURISH IT.[2]

- It can be found in our skin, bones, nerves, muscles, cells, digestive and reproductive system.

- Protects the genes in the body which help to repair DNA in body cells.

- Fluoride in toothpaste/water destroys melanin production in the pineal gland.

- Melanin is able to take energy in the form of light and transfer it into a usable source of energy in the body as food (nutrients.)

- We have 360 melanin centers in our stomach/less melanated people have forty.[2] That dark line on the stomach when a black woman becomes pregnant is from increased melanin production to protect the baby from ultraviolet rays.[2]

- The melanin centers in the stomach allow for greater metabolization of food due to the live bacteria that dwell in our gastrointestinal tract (aids digestion).

- Melanin is a molecule that broadcasts and receives information by way of light and sound frequencies.

- Melanin is a neurochemical produced by our pineal gland (third eye) near the center of our brain. The pineal gland resembles a pine cone and is about the size of a pea.

- Melanin metabolizes carbohydrates, slows aging, strengthens the immune system, and boosts memory.

- Melanin is an intelligent free radical (cell damaging) protector. Melanin acts as a deposit site for unpaired electrons, which removes free radicals.

- It allows the African man to have the highest level of testosterone. [3]

The blacker the berry the sweeter the juice is pure facts. Black skin ages approximately ten years slower than less melanated skin. Why would you not love your blackness? You're hiding from the sun, trying to reduce your melanin, while others are trying to roast in the sun to increase their melanin to become you. Individuals with black or brown eyes have more melanin to block the sun rays. Those with blue, green or hazel have little melanin/protection from the sun and can experience more irritation and discomfort without eye protection. I know a lot of people with brown eyes would love to have hazel or green, but love those beautiful brown eyes and know you are protected.

It is presumed that scientists do not fully understand the function of neuromelanin (melanin in the brain). We have African doctors sharing the critical function of melanin in our brains, but the information is not being published on a large scale.

"As you section the brain, the deeper you go; the more melanin you see."[4] Dr. Ann Brown tells us that two scientists did a mapping of the brain and located twelve centers in the African man that contain Eumelanin. Europeans have two centers in their brain, which makes them more prone to neurological disease. The twelve centers are responsible for allowing your brain to transmit and receive information at a higher rate than any other race.

There are three types of melanin: eumelanin, pheomelanin, and neuromelanin. Cells in the skin that produce and secrete melanin are called melanocytes. Melanocytes are found between the cells of the epidermis and can change from the natural aging process or direct stimulation. Eumelanin and pheomelanin play key roles in eye, hair, and skin color. Pheomelanin is the chemical responsible for blonde and red hair, lighter skin tones, and green and blue eyes. Pheomelanin reflects energy, and this is the reason white people can't stand in the sun for long periods of time. European people are primarily pheomelanin dominant, which is obvious once you see a pinkish pigmentation. Eumelanin is the complete opposite and has the ability to absorb and store energy. The more energy absorbed, the darker the melanin. Melanin is jet black in its purest form.

The brain doesn't produce eumelanin, so we need to eat foods that contain pigment to produce it in order to replenish those twelve centers in the brain. What foods have pigment? Natural foods – food that you can find in nature; not in aisle seven in the supermarket, next to the Frosted Flakes. When the food metabolizes, the natural pigment in the foods regenerate any cells in the body that are damaged. It is important to consume as much natural foods as possible to decrease the risk of neurological diseases. Over accumulation of toxic-unnatural substances absorbed by neuromelanin overtime can lead to cellular damage.

Studies have shown that people of color have a lower prevalence of Alzheimer's and Parkinson's disease due to the high level of brain melanin. That brain melanin is an antioxidant that prevents damage to the cells. Many drugs used to treat mental disease such as these two, adversely affect the brain's (melanated centers) ability to transmit messages in our body.

"THE DARKER THE FLESH THEN THE DEEPER THE ROOTS"

We are the only community that has veered so left from the diet of our ancestors. Orientals and Indians have a longer life span because they stick to their traditional ancestral diet. Orientals and Indians know that the western standard of medicine cannot benefit their people and that's why they have their own medical system based on their biological make-up. Our melanin needs natural foods with pigment that you'll find in chapter fifteen. This decreases our chance of degenerative disease in the brain and other organs in our bodies. Toxins accumulate in the body from high consumption of unnatural fats, meats, tap water, drugs and alcohol to be absorbed by the melanin in our bodies. Now we have cell damage that causes a host of problems like dis-ease and fast aging.

Our slavery went deep beyond the physical during the Transatlantic Slave Trade. It is mental, and the easiest way to attack your mental, physical and spiritual well-being is through your diet. Europeans took away your spirituality and gave you religion. They took away true education and gave you indoctrination. They took away your high plant protein diet with minimal starches and gave you pork belly and white rice.

You may not know it, but the food is attacking your soul. Altering the melanin through food will alter your brain. Toxic diet + Toxic thinking = debilitating health. Europeans introduced their engineered, poisonous foods to you because they knew destroying your bodies would limit your overall capabilities.

IT'S IN YOUR SOUL

Melanin goes deep beyond the mind and body; it is your soul. You are the most influential race and get no credit for it. You create and others copy/steal. Can we all agree that more than a majority of African/ Hispanic people move differently than any other race? You walk different, you talk different… you have what we like to call swag. Swag is a natural rhythm that is instilled in you from birth or even before birth.

Brothers, that creativity that you naturally have to spit 16 bars off the top is your melanin. Sisters your spontaneous creativity, how you dance, your intuition… that's all melanin. When you're introduced to someone new and you have a good or bad "vibe," that's the pineal gland picking up energy. Melanin helps you pick up on what your five senses can't by allowing you access to a higher form of energy.

There is a circadian (rhythm) in our bodies governed by the pineal gland that secretes hormones at night (melatonin) and hormones during the day (serotonin) to keep you balanced. Essentially, it's our wake and sleep patterns. Melatonin also keeps the digestive cycle in balance as long as you aren't eating food from morning to late hours in the night. The rhythm of the digestive process is controlled by the pineal glands ability to function so it is very important to nurture it.

RATED-PG

The pineal gland is often referred to as the "principal seat of our soul, and the place in which all our thoughts are formed." The ancients have deemed it as a connection between the physical and spiritual world. It's the inner space that gives you access to the outer space. Also known as the third eye, it works in connection with our hypothalamus gland which is responsible for our thirst, hunger, sexual desire, and the biological clock that determines our aging.

The pineal gland is in the third ventricle and sits at the end of stalks of neurons called the habenula stalk. Its ability to function is disturbed when the body is living off processed, bleached, junk food. These "foods" disrupt your ability to control yourself because all the nutrients have been taken out of the foods which causes the pineal gland to become underactive. Melanin is produced primarily by our pineal gland and that gland activates responses in all the other glands in our body to keep the body in harmony.

All races have melanin, but the capacity to interact with the universe is limited to those with more melanin. According to John Hopkins University, there are six race classes:

- 6 – Africans/Black (highest melanin content)

- 5 – Black/Brown (Mexican, Malaysian, Native Indians, Hispanic)

- 4 – Red (Native American, Japanese)

- 2-3 – Yellow (Oriental)

- 1 – Caucasian (lowest melanin content)[5]

Africans are rated the highest in respect to our melanin content. Melanin is not taken into consideration when we get our bloodwork from the doctor. Our uniqueness is being hidden from us, so we have to do the work ourselves to maintain our heath. Dr. Afrika makes an interesting point about bloodwork that I'll summarize here. There are times where you may not feel well, so you go to the doctor. They take bloodwork and tell you that you're fine. The reason you still feel dis-ease, even though the bloodwork shows the opposite is because the tests are based on a European person's blood content.

"You being at their normal level means you're twice as sick. Melanin causes you to need more vitamins and minerals in your body than any other race."[6] Black people get diabetes with glucose levels in the normal range for white people. It's due to our higher melanin con-tent, which makes us more susceptible to diabetes from the same sugar intake as a person with the least melanin. Your baby's formula is based on a European woman's breast milk as opposed to a woman of color's. The breast milk of black women has a higher nutrient content. People of African descent have 10x more bone density than Caucasians so using their standard for measuring bone density is dangerous.

Dr. Jewel Pookrum shared with us in her lecture on, "*Differences between Africans and other races and cell generation*," that the National Medical Association published in an article in 1975 that said, "There are lifelong differences in hemoglobin levels between blacks and whites."[7] Still to this day, the values of Caucasian bloodwork is used as a standard for people of color.

She also tells us that Dr. Stanley Garn (Caucasian doctor) of the University of Michigan submitted this information to the Black Medical Association and they did nothing with it. Doctors in the Western world are taught in medical school to use the standard test, which is based on a Caucasians person's blood value. The melanin deficiency in European people as the basis for blood work affects our vitamin levels and our overall health.

Over 80%, of our diseases are from what we put in our mouth and breathe through our lungs. Our problem is medical science is treating the symptoms and not the causes. Melanin is an amazing component given to black/brown people and you will learn in this book how to treat it.

HOW COME THEY HAVE ON SHORTS IN THE WINTER?

This is something I've always wondered about Caucasian people. Why the hell are they jogging in twenty degrees with shorts on? Dr. Jewel Pookrum explains it perfectly in her lecture about melanin.

Black people do not have a circulatory system to support a cold environment. Due to our high melanin content, we have to have blood in two places at the same time. We have to have blood under the skin to feed the second brain due to all the melanin. The second place of supply is needed deep within our organs. White people can play hockey, ski, jog in shorts in the snow, all cold activities because they hold all their blood supply deep in their body's organs. They don't feel cold because they don't have all the blood supply taking a lot of information to their skin.[8] What Dr. Pookrum is saying is that pigmented neurons in the nervous system and melanocytes in the skin have the same origin; that's why she refers to the skin as the second brain.

Lastly, European people have a higher amount of sulfur and ammonia present in their melanin. Black people are higher in selenium with minimal sulfur because we are eumelanin dominant. Ammonia warms up in a cold environment, so that is also why most white people aren't affected by inclement weather. Internally, we have different chemistry.

THE HUMAN PLANT

I truly believe the lack of familiarity with our body systems is what causes us to neglect our bodies. Long before chemicals were manufactured in labs to make medicine, whole plants were used for healing. The similarity between plants and human are remarkable.

My uncle Vern used to grow marijuana plants and after his first go around of killing the entire garden I realized that the plants basic necessities are similar to melanin dominant people. Plants need carbon, hydrogen and oxygen, which are absorbed from air and water. Ninety percent of humans are made of these exact elements. The rest of the nutrients plants need to maintain health are absorbed through the soil. Nutrients such as nitrogen, potassium, magnesium, zinc, and phosphorus are able to transfer from one section of the plant to another. The nutrients move to the specific part of the plant where they are needed. This is so similar to humans because the melanin travels to the area of the body that is deficient or weak and in need of tissue repair/regeneration.

Magnesium is the central atom in every chlorophyll molecule, and like melanin magnesium is needed to take sunlight and transfer it into usable energy. It also neutralizes toxic waste produced by the plants or in the soil. Melanin can neutralize harmful free radicals and radiation. Melanin and magnesium aid in the utilization of nutrients such as carbohydrates into the body. A melanin deficiency is common in the western world due to lack of sunlight for half of the year. A magnesium deficiency is common for indoor plants leaving the leaves rusty and discolored. Plants and melanin dominant individuals need sunlight for optimal health.

Nitrogen is also one of the most important element required for plant growth. It regulates the marijuana plants ability to make proteins in the cells, producing amino acids and chlorophyll, and it's responsible for stem and leaf growth. The presence of melanin is responsible for the growth of hair, bones, and overall development in humans. Nitrogen is a common nutrient deficiency in plants and causes: the leaves to lose its luster, yellow leaves, weak stems, slow root development and interveinal chlorosis (yellow between the veins) eventually causing the leaf to die and drop off. An abnormal amount of melanin at the time of conception can cause neurological defects and retardation to the unborn baby.

YOU FEEL ME?

Dr. Sebi refers to us as electric people. Electricity is found throughout the human body and allows us to have signals sent from the nervous system to body. This is why we can think, feel, and move. Without electricity, you wouldn't be reading this book right now. Our body depends on electrical signals because with only chemical signals, we wouldn't be able to respond in an instance.

If we are walking in the woods and a bear is chasing us, it's the electric impulse plus the chemical reaction in our body that would tell us to run. Electricity allows our cells to communicate with each other. When you get in touch with your pineal gland, you will understand the true meaning of energy and vibrations. There is an electromagnetic force field inside your brain underneath your pineal gland that gives you access to different levels of consciousness. Melanin generates current for impulse transmission between cells.

Raw natural foods transfer their energy into the body cells. As we learned from the law of conservation, energy is neither created nor destroyed, it can only be transferred or changed from one form to another. Processed cooked food has little to no energy which we can all see for ourselves when we have an anti-nutritious meal. It leaves us feeling depleted of all our energy reserves. Raw foods such as plants have a high vibration and give us high energy levels. Energy between all living things become one, therefore plant and man become one. So instead of rotting in the ground, a plant wants to become a part of another life form.

If we have a healthy body and a poisoned mind, we will be sick. If we have a healthy mind and a poisoned body, we will be sick. The goal is to have a balance between the two, so what I want to do here is give you a new medical system. This is the system called **prevention**, that doesn't seem to exist in Western medicine. To the medical society, you are more revenue for research than human beings. I hope you're ready to become your own healer in a society that has created and monetized your ignorance and sickness.

**Always remember, you won't be provided with
the truth when the lie is more profitable.**

1. Afrika, Laila O. The Power and Science of Melanin; The Biochemical that makes black people black; pg. 5

2. Dr. Laila O. Afrika. Published January 22, 2014. Understanding Melanin. https://youtube.com/watch?v=SO0Ri7PEdQcandfeature=youtu.be

3. Brown, Ann. Published on December 17, 2012. "Melanin & Pineal Gland pt. 1." https://youtu.be/qYTfR60XsFU

4. Afrika, Laila O. The Power and Science of Melanin; The Biochemical that makes black people black; pg. 5

5. Afrika, Laila O Published January 22, 2014. Understanding Melanin. https://youtube.com/watch?v=SO0Ri7PEdQcandfeature=youtu.be

6. 7. 8. Pookrum, Jewel. Published March 24, 2016. "Differences between Africans and other races and cell regeneration." https://youtu.be/yJIF6BYS9po

2

MELANIN MANIPULATION

"Among the Egyptians themselves, those who dwell in the cultivated country are the most careful of all men to preserve the memory of the past, and none of whom I have questioned have so many chronicles…

**For there are three consecutive days in every month
they purge themselves, pursuing after health by means
of emetics and drenches; for they think it is from the
food which they eat that all sickness come to men."**

–ANCIENT EGYPTIAN PROVERB

Our ancient Egyptian ancestors knew that the cure to all ailments, aches, pain and overall dis-ease are provided by nature. They knew dis-ease comes from poor diet practices. In this current day and age, with fast/over-processed food everywhere we turn in our community, highly melanated people are experiencing debilitating health and have nowhere to turn. We have to work on going back to our original diet prior to slavery.

"From 1984 to 1989 life expectancy for whites increased, while life expectancy for blacks decreased."[9] We can attribute part of the statistics to upbringing, lifestyle and diet. Growing up in East Flatbush, Brooklyn, New York, on every corner there's a Wendy's, McDonalds, Chinese restaurant, Kennedys Fried chicken etc. Supermarkets are overflowing with aisles of processed food, non-organic meat, farm-raised fish, and non-organic vegetables and fruits.

Then on the flip side, take a drive over to Park Slope, Ft. Greene, or Ditmas Park; there are organic supermarkets, healthy restaurants, vitamin shops, and a plethora of juice bars.

It's no surprise that major cities throughout the Unites States are organized by racial groups. The obvious racial organization in America is due to the segregation and unconstitutional racial zoning enforced by government. In *"The Color of Law: A forgotten history of how Government Segregated America,"* Richard Rothstein presents the long history of federal, state and local policy that produced a well-organized segregation all across America.[10] I am by no means saying that integration would have saved our communities, but having access to better housing, schools, and food options would have been crucial to communities of color thriving in America. It is quite clear that this was not the main objective that white America had for our kings and queens.

Think about the feeling you have after a large plate of white rice, pork chops, fried chicken, mac 'n cheese, and a cup of juice. You develop what we call in urban neighborhoods, "the itis." This type of food, if you can even call it food, requires energy to metabolize in the body. The energy comes from other organ systems which helps increase the blood supply to the stomach to help break the food down. This is what causes a fatigued feeling after eating. Real nutritious foods don't give you that sleepy, drained feeling.

The "itis" is what's clouding our minds and holding us back from our true awakening as a whole, to start solving the issues that affect our community. From the inception of colonization, Europeans suppressed our melanin because they knew the power of fueling our bodies with quality food, which would enhance our minds and enlighten our souls. Europeans fed us poison during slavery which we now call "Soul food." "But good for whose soul?" [11]

The nutritional plantation has been used to replace the physical plantation because controlling your mind is way more powerful than controlling your body.

My goal in this section of *We Are Not the Same*, is to present you with several options for cleansing your amazing bodies, starting with the most efficient, yet stringent way to reset your digestive system. It makes sense to first understand a little about how our digestive system works. This will allow us to see why it's in our best interest to reduce or eliminate our intake of processed foods, white flour, sugar, "chopped cheese", excess salt and flesh foods. Your melanin and your immune system are in an intimate relationship until they are disrupted by poor diet and toxic environment. Under the skin, people of color are different and have to be treated as such.

DIGESTION

The process of digestion begins once we smell food. That smell stimulates the digestive organs to get ready. This is why when you see food you say, "my mouth is watering." You are now ready for those digestive enzymes to mix with the food you're about to eat. Saliva is not just a clear liquid; it is actually chemistry going on in your mouth to break down foods. This is why chewing your food properly is so important.

When my family would get together to have dinner, my brother would pray with one eye open, waiting to devour what lay before him, while making sure no one went near his plate. It was like a race that involved gulping and not enough chewing. The salivary enzyme that helps break down food is called amylase. This enzyme is only effective when food is chewed to completion. It cannot breakdown fats and proteins, only carbohydrates into simpler form.

Food that is not chewed to completion travels through our esophagus then into our stomach to be left undigested. Our stomachs are not equipped to break down large chunks of food. So, for all of my fast eating brothers and sisters out there, please take your time and chew your food. Put down those weapons called a knife and fork between bites.

The stomach produces hydrochloric acid and the enzyme pepsin, which turns the food into chyme and makes it a paste-like consistency. Proteins like chicken and steak need the acidic environment from the stomach to be broken down. The liquid is then passed through the duodenum to be saturated with digestive fluids from the pancreas and liver. As you can see in the sketch below, that paste travels through a twenty-five foot or so coiled tube called the small intestine, all neatly packed in our midsection.

The small intestine is where the vitamins and nutrients from our liquefied food are reduced to a chemical substance to be absorbed into the bloodstream. Waste left over from the digestive process is passed through the large intestine (colon) until a mass movement empties it into the rectum, hopefully one to three times a day. Think about how many of us actually do "number two" daily. The stool passed into the toilet is mostly left over food debris and bacteria. On average, it takes about thirty to forty hours for stool to get through the colon.

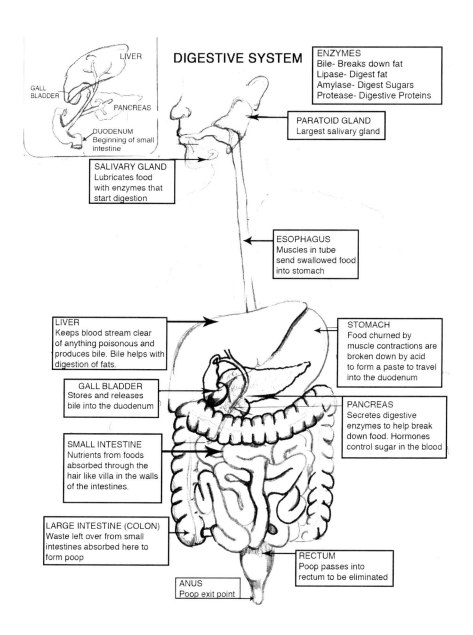

DIGESTIVE SYSTEM

LIVER

GALL BLADDER

PANCREAS

DUODENUM
Beginning of small intestine

ENZYMES
Bile- Breaks down fat
Lipase- Digest fat
Amylase- Digest Sugars
Protease- Digestive Proteins

PARATOID GLAND
Largest salivary gland

SALIVARY GLAND
Lubricates food with enzymes that start digestion

ESOPHAGUS
Muscles in tube send swallowed food into stomach

LIVER
Keeps blood stream clear of anything poisonous and produces bile. Bile helps with digestion of fats.

STOMACH
Food churned by muscle contractions are broken down by acid to form a paste to travel into the duodenum

GALL BLADDER
Stores and releases bile into the duodenum

PANCREAS
Secretes digestive enzymes to help break down food. Hormones control sugar in the blood

SMALL INTESTINE
Nutrients from foods absorbed through the hair like villa in the walls of the intestines.

LARGE INTESTINE (COLON)
Waste left over from small intestines absorbed here to form poop

RECTUM
Poop passes into rectum to be eliminated

ANUS
Poop exit point

Such an arduous process is done by our bodies effortlessly, but unfortunately, when there isn't a well-balanced diet to assist with carrying out this seamless operation things get quite constipated... I mean complicated. If our diet lacks fiber and consists mostly of goat, rice and peas, mac 'n cheese... you get my drift – these highly refined foods can lead to compaction of waste in the colon; allowing waste that should be excreted to be absorbed back into the body. In layman's terms, your shit is reversing back up your colon into your small intestines.

Constipation is caused by improperly masticated food whose waste matter is left in the body too long. When food hangs out in your system too long, peristaltic contractions in your digestive tract may be decreased. All this compaction of mucoid (mucus that traps toxins in the intestine) and matter cling to the walls of the colon. Improper functioning of the digestive system can lead to headaches, brain fog, allergies, dry skin, and in extreme cases, cancer.

Your colon can be thought of as a drain pipe in your toilet bowl. When your drain is clogged and you try to flush the toilet the waste backs up and spills all over your bathroom floor. When this happens to our colon, the waste spills over into another important filter called our lymphatic system.

Lymph is a clear fluid containing cells that flows throughout different channels in our body, collecting impurities such as bacteria, old red blood cells, cellular waste, heavy metals, pesticides, and drug residue. This fluid circulates around the body through muscle movement. This is why being physically active is crucial. When that lymph fluid makes a stop in the lymph nodes, which you can feel in your neck, armpits, or groin area, those nodes destroy whatever impurities are being carried through your body.

If you have a lymph node in any of those areas that is enlarged, that means the toxins are too much and you need to stop whatever you're doing and cleanse. You can think of the lymph node as the dump site for toxin collection. If these two areas are getting backed up, the waste travels back into our bloodstream. That is essentially what disease is, waste being reabsorbed back into the body due to poor digestion, assimilation and elimination.

Now that we know a little about how our amazing bodies excrete waste, let us look into several ways in which we can assist our bodies in taking a much-needed break. The first of many options to cleanse is called fasting.

FASTING

"Salvation is the freeing of the soul from its bodily fetters; becoming God through knowledge and wisdom; controlling the forces of the cosmos instead of being a slave to them; Subduing the lower nature and through awakening the higher self, ending the cycle of rebirth and dwelling with the Neters who direct and control the Great Plan"

-ANCIENT EGYPTIAN PROVERB

Every living thing produces waste which they must get rid of or it will interfere with the process of life. Fasting is a physiological vacation which has been practiced for over 10,000 years. It is an amazing practice that can heal almost any dis-ease and the best part is, IT'S FREE! The most difficult situation that arises in a fast is what goes on in our mind and gaining control over our thoughts and not being a slave to them; thus being weakened as our ancestors mentioned. Physical and mental preparation for the side effects are key, so slowly ease yourself in.

In a fast, we would abstain from all foods and drink only water. Wait, don't close the book yet. I will provide more options once this lesson is complete. During a water fast, your digestive system is no longer occupied with the strenuous task of constant food processing and elimination. Now it can focus all of its energy on elimination of fat stores, dissolve dis-ease deposits from deep tissues, cysts, tumors, abscesses, ulcers, and any other non-beneficial foreigners invading our bodies.

I like to call these unwanted foreigners colonizers. These colonizers are what's interrupting the regular function of our eliminatory systems. Name one situation in history where allowing foreigners to invade/occupy any space has benefited native occupants. I'm drawing a blank as well, but I digress.

If we don't take eliminating poisons out of our systems seriously, the poisons will eliminate us; which is all traced back to white supremacy and racism to eliminate black and brown people in all areas of the system. Which system you might ask? Dr. Frances Cress Welsing said it best in the *Cress theory lecture* where she explained, Racism is a system of destruction of nonwhite people in all areas not limited to economics, education, labor, entertainment, law, politics, religion and sex.[12]

To that list I would like to add nutrition… Nutritional Racism. Melanated people need to understand the power of a pure body and the affects it has on mental, physical and spiritual power. "Take away food from a sick man's stomach and you have begun, not to starve the sick man, but the disease."[13]

The liver and kidneys are so burdened with eliminating unnatural substances that it stores these toxins in the weakest tissues in an effort to preserve the integrity of the blood. For examples, if it's stored in the joints it's called arthritis, pancreas- diabetes, blood- high blood pressure, etc.

WHAT HAPPENS TO YOUR BODY DURING A FAST?

Fasting is a curative element that can bring the body back to balance. There is an interesting process that happens to your body during a water fast. Your body begins to live on its reserves. Even for the skinniest dis-eased person, a fast is beneficial because we all have reserves for our body to eliminate. The intelligent mechanism performed by our body is called autolysis, which simply means to self-digest. Your body literally begins living off the toxins or weak areas in your body to begin the healing process.

Think about when you have a basic cold, fever or flu and you lose your appetite. What does mom usually suggest? Eat some food to get some energy. Sorry mom, that's the complete opposite of what we should be doing. We need to adhere to nature's laws. Meaning, if your body doesn't want food, then don't give it food because it wants to clear your dis-ease without any interruptions. Melanin dominant individuals have the ability to heal themselves in half the time compared to melanin recessive people. Every function performed by the human body is done through information being processed by the brain except for melanin. **Melanin acts independently which means it processes its own information and travels to where it is needed in the body.**

I'm not going to lie; I myself have performed several water fasts ranging from one to ten days and the beginning is extremely difficult, even for the mentally strong. You will feel symptoms that you will confuse with hunger, but I can assure it's the complete opposite of hunger. It's your body pushing years and years of toxins, uric acid, mucus, and prescription drugs out of your body through the bloodstream and finally through all avenues of excretion.

The poisons that have been locked up in your systems for many years have broken loose and are running a riot in your blood like Nat Turner during a slave rebellion. "Drugs taken ten, twenty, thirty, and even forty years ago were expelled together with mucus. I had obese patients that eliminated from their body as much as fifty to sixty pounds of waste, and one – fifteen pounds alone from the colon – mainly consisting of foreign matters, especially old, hardened, feces."[14]

The chemicals in prescription drugs disrupt the normal balance of the cells which leads to their destruction. Western medicine likes to call the disruption of the normal cells along with the dis-eased cells from medication, "side effects." That is because synthetic drugs run through the healthy and sick cells causing further complications later on down the line.

Symptoms that can be expected within the first two to three days of the fast are as follows:

- Headaches and dizziness

- Eruptions on the skin

- Vomiting

- Heavily coated tongue (white, yellow or black – the darker the more toxic you are). What you would call "hunger breath" is toxins being released after not eating for a certain amount of time. Now you know why your breath is hot ☺

- Hunger pangs in the stomach. (This is not true hunger)

- Discharge of excess mucus through the mouth, nose, lungs, vagina or penis

- Slight weakness

These symptoms are referred to as "the healing crisis" during a fast. Your body is attempting to eliminate toxins faster than the elimination paths can remove them. This is the reason I always suggest daily coffee enemas along with fasting to assist with the symptoms and proper elimination of waste. More on coffee enemas in chapter twelve.

In traditional African medicine, the tongue mirrors the intestines, so even if you brush your tongue or use a tongue scraper, you will not be able to remove the coating (toxins) off your tongue until the poisons pass through your body, or the fast has ended. Your tongue shows you what is happening inside your body and this is exactly what happened to myself and my colleagues when the fast was performed.

It is truly amazing to see the interconnectedness of our bodies; which simply means everything is connected to everything and communicates through energy (also known as "chi" in Chinese medicine). The energy comes from an area in the cell called mitochondria. Look at mitochondria as the power plant of cells. Drugs, pesticides, mercury from dental fillings leaking into the body, contaminated water, households, chemicals etc. disrupts the energy conductor throughout the body cells and causes a "brownout". Natural foods and herbs help repair the brownout between the cells allowing for a seamless flow of energy.

Dis-ease prevention is solely dependent on the cell's ability to self-repair and regenerate. Properly nourished melanin helps to repair defective cells. Defective cells don't know how to stop multiplying; they don't have a programmed cell death.

There is no need to separate organs and name diseases when they are all caused by the same thing. Food, drugs, alcohol, smoking, tap water, negative thoughts, stress, and environmental toxins.

Where was I? Oh yes, fasting. Don't give up on me until you hear the positive aspects of the fast which far outweigh the discomforts.

Herbert M. Shelton says, "Regeneration of the body is a ceaseless process. The daily renewal of its cells and tissues prevents old age and early death for considerable time, despite the worst abuses which are heaped upon the bodies of most of us."[15]

Some results to expect from the fast depending on the length are:

- A return of the whites (sclera) in the eyes

- Clearing up of pimples and blotches on the skin (rejuvenated blood)

- Strengthens the heart (removes heavy load from the heart)

- Elimination of toxins from decomposed foods in the digestive tract

- Mental clarity and power increased

- Weight loss

- Improved testosterone levels and sperm count

- Dissolved cysts or fibroids in the uterus/ Dissolved cysts in the prostate gland

- Joint pain relief (Joint pain caused by inorganic deposits that settle between the joints and lack of circulation of the blood in certain areas where you feel aches and pain are now freed up)

Aside from the amazing benefits listed above, I also want to include the reversal of asthma which is affecting a lot of people of color. The reversal of asthma was proven a number of times by Upton Sinclair's

"*The Fasting Cure*" which includes a myriad of letters of patients writing to him about their dis-ease being reversed.

The skin eliminates dead cells naturally, unless your body is in such a dis-eased state that your pores are clogged and suffocating with decayed matter. Are you the type of person or do you know someone who can squeeze their nose and a bunch of tiny, worm-looking particles squirt out? Yes? That's not normal and you need to be cleansed. Baths are highly recommended during the fast to eliminate waste from the skin.

The body gets rid of carbon dioxide from the lungs, fecal matter from the intestines, urine from the kidneys, and sweat from the skin. The process of elimination is just as important as the process of ingestion.

If this is your first time fasting, I would recommend trying a sixteen to twenty-four hour fast, which is very beneficial for your digestive tract, as it rids your body of toxins. Once you have conquered that several times, you can go on an extended fast; the length of time depends on what your goals are. For general house cleaning, two to three days a month or seasonal fasts are great! For a particular dis-ease, usually one to four weeks can assist in expelling the cause of the dis-ease, but the fast has to be monitored by a professional. For optimal detoxification in the cells, 72-84 hours of fasting is recommended. For myself the third day was the roughest. Once you get passed the third day the hunger and symptoms slowly dissipate.

When I comb my hair, the weak, unnourished strands fall out first. The same thing happens in the body; the weak particles cannot survive a fast and will be combed out through your elimination points. Please be aware that if you return to a degenerate lifestyle and begin consuming garbage on a regular basis, the dis-ease will return. Nutrition and life are all about balance.

People who know me really well always ask me if I'm having grass for dinner and the answer is usually yes (LOL). I do have what society calls "cheat meals" and they are far more enjoyable when you have them once in a while as opposed to daily. Trust me!

Ending the fast is very important and is not something that shouldn't be rushed. The key is to have easy to digest foods after the fast has ended. You can break your fast with either fruits or vegetables. By doing this, you can continue the cleansing of your intestinal lining and the waste can keep moving. Typically, once you break the fast with fruits, you will have a bowel movement right away. This is because your body has softened up the decayed matter that has been sitting there that has now been loosened from the absence of food.

Once you've reintroduced yourself to fresh juices or raw fruits and veggies, you can now add in steamed low starch veggies such as spinach, kale, yams etc. Take half of your cleansing regimen time to return to your diet. If you did a one-week fast, it should take you approximately three days to return to your diet with a healthier approach.

If you still want to attempt a water fast, but twenty-four hours is too drastic, you also have the option of **intermittent fasting** which also has great benefits. Instead of eating between the hours of 7am and 9pm, or whatever hours you're used to having breakfast, lunch, and dinner, you would eat all meals within eight hours. The optimal time for eating is between the hours of 12pm and 7pm with the heaviest meal being consumed between 1pm and 3pm. I practice intermittent fasting all year round.

Remember that with regular fasting and change of diet, it will take years for the mass quantities of toxins that have accumulated over your lifespan to be completely removed from the body. You will still notice a change very soon once you start. Healing also depends greatly on mental attitudes, so stay positive.

Warning: Certain prescription drugs cannot be stopped abruptly in order to attempt a water fast; they require you to be weaned off overtime. Please verify fasting or change in diet with your physician. Diabetics should fast only under a health care professional's supervision.

9. Walker, Marcellus A. M.D and Singleton, Kenneth B., M.D. *Natural Health for African Americans*, New York, (February 1999), pg.3

10. Rothstein, Richard. *The Color of Law*: A Forgotten History of How Our Government Segregated America. First edition. New York: Liveright Publishing Corporation, 2017.

11. Dr. Laila O. Afrika. Published January 22, 2014. *"Understanding Melanin."* https://youtube.com/watch?v=SO0Ri7PEdQcandfeature=youtu.be

12. Welsing, Frances Cress. *The Isis Papers: The key to colors*. C.W. Publishing, Washington D.C. 1991

13. Macfadden, Bernarr. *Fasting- Hydrotherapy Nature Exercise;* Natures Wonderful Remedies for the Cure; Dp all Acute. Published by The Physical Culture Publishing Co. Originally published 1900, pg.15

14. Ehret, Arnold, Annotated, Revised, and Edited by Prof. Spira Prof. Arnold Ehret's. *Mucusless Diet Healing System* Revised, (November 2015), pg.17

15. Shelton, Herbert M. *The Science and Fine Arts of Fasting*. Published by Dr. Shelton's Health School, (Fourth revised edition 1963), pg. 213

3

"SIPPIN' ON GIN AND JUICE"

JUICE DIET

Juice diets are also extremely beneficial for the healing of the Melanated body. The only gin you should be sippin' on is ginger shots accompanied with a green juice. I say juice diet because the true meaning of "fast" is to abstain from solid foods, surviving on water alone for several days.

Juice diets are instrumental in assisting the body with clearing out the organs of elimination and allowing for easy absorption of vitamins and minerals, without calling in excess help from our digestive system. Organs of elimination are the skin, the lymphatic system, kidneys, lungs, large and small intestines, and liver. I will cover the liver in a separate section, due to the love of Hennessey by our community.

In a typical juice diet, you would drink anywhere from four to six juices a day depending on your individual needs. Similar to the fast, your body will still remove toxins. You will have more energy, clearing up of the skin, and mental clarity. I highly recommend organic cold-pressed, raw fruit and vegetable juice. A cold-pressed juicer is more efficient than a centrifugal juicer in extracting the juice from the veggies and fruits while retaining the important nutrients and enzymes to be assimilated into your bloodstream.

Our body creates new cells every thirty-five days based on the foods/drinks that we consume, so even if you're not ready for a water fast, a juice diet is a great start to reset your system. At the end of this section, you will find a couple juice recipes to prepare at home or you can always go to your local, organic juice bar.

Remember, while your body is releasing foreign materials from your cells, you will feel symptoms in the weakened, overburdened areas in your body. Eventually the symptoms will fade and cell regeneration will begin.

Organic fruits and vegetables would be my first choice because they tend to have less pesticide residue than non-organic. Organic fruits and vegetables are not grown with synthetic or chemical fertilizer, thus enhancing your vitamin and antioxidant intake by about 20-40%.

By the definition provided by the National Institute of Environmental Health Sciences, a pesticide is any substance used to kill, repel, or control certain forms of plant or animal life that are considered pests. Simply put, pesticides are poisons that affect our health over time with exposure. The effects of ingesting pesticides can range from a simple sore throat, headache, or cough to asthma, Parkinson's disease or cancer. If the cost of organic fruits and veggies are out of your budget, still incorporate regular fruits and veggies in your diet; just wash the hell out of them. "It's fifteen times better to eat the commercially-grown, non-organic produce than it is to avoid fruit and vegetables just because they've been sprayed."[16]

For beginners, I would recommend a juice diet starting at twenty-four hours and once you have mastered that, you can increase it from two to seven days. These diets are good to perform once or twice a month to give our elimination systems a much needed break. Or you can have one liquid day weekly. To enhance nutrient absorption, take a digestive enzyme twenty minutes prior to drinking juices.

Remember, the main purpose of juicing is to concentrate the nutrients and make them easily digestible by the body.

Example Juice Combinations:

Wash and prep your organic fruits and veggies!!!

- **Green Detox**: Kale, celery, 5pcs of parsley, 1 inch of burdock root, watercress, ½ an apple, ½ lime and 1inch ginger

- **Beginner Greens**: One apple, ½ beet, one carrot, handful of spinach and kale, ½ lime

- **Smooth skin Green Juice**: One cucumber, four to six celery ribs, two handfuls of kale and watercress, ½ lime, and 1in ginger

- **Pick me up**: Two medium beets, one Granny Smith apple, two carrots, and 1tbsp. of chia seeds (optional). Chia seeds are great for an extra fiber kick and contain plant-based protein.

*I don't have precise measurements for the greens because I tend to make mine bitter. Try out a few different measurements but don't make it too sweet.

RAW FOOD DIET

I learned about the benefits of raw food diets roughly ten years ago when I found myself becoming sick every month and going to the hospital for care several times throughout 2008. My blood test results came back inconclusive every time. Maybe it's because the lab work isn't based on the values of a person of color. Or it could be that blood work in Western medicine is based on the values of sick people. If you aren't sick enough, chances are they won't be able to give you a proper diagnosis until you're far along into your dis-ease.

I came across research from an amazing herbalist named Dr. Sebi who promoted raw and natural foods for the true healing of our bodies, and not self-medicating, which only masks the symptoms while causing more issues. From March to June, My friend Rubskin and I performed the raw food diet with herbal supplements provided by a company called Dherbs, and the results were amazing!

The reason I didn't use Dr. Sebi's products was because they were way out of my budget at the time. After more research, I found Dherbs, which I believe gave me the same results Dr. Sebi's cleanse would have. I had glowing skin and my ailments the doctor couldn't detect disappeared. I lost fifteen pounds, which wasn't the reason for doing the diet and my joint issues in my knees went away.

Raw foods are a great detox; it just works a little slower than water fasting or juicing. I was only twenty-six with these issues, so clearly it was my terrible diet breaking my body down until I couldn't take it anymore.

I truly believe, as advanced as science is, everything cannot be detected through medical science and there are some things we have to know, feel and believe for ourselves. We must listen to our bodies, despite what the doctor is saying. I am NOT saying to avoid the doctor, because people of color (especially men) statistically do not go to the doctor until are sick. What I'm saying is, go to the doctor annually for check-ups, but become your own physician at home. Initiate the process we're calling prevention.

To perform this Raw Food Diet, eliminate all flesh, dairy and cooked foods from your diet. The idea is the same as with fasting and juicing; give your body the rest it needs from breaking down and trying to eliminate the over processed foods in our bodies. You can only eat fruits, nuts and vegetables in their natural state. Raw foods digest more easily than cooked and pass through the system quicker, taking no time to decompose in the colon.

The way I made this fun was going out to eat at raw food restaurants which prepare foods in such a creative and healthy way through the process of dehydration. Dehydration is a process in which you "cook" food between 105F/41C and 115F/46C. Raw food experts believe that once you cook food at 118F and higher, you're destroying the vitamins and enzymes needed from food that are essential to our health. The basic function of enzymes is to break down proteins and starches. If your diet consist of primarily cooked foods above 140F/60C issues such as constipation, diarrhea, gas pains and poor digestion usually occur. I believe that once we do monthly or at least seasonal house cleaning of our bodies, we can still enjoy cooked foods from time to time without it being detrimental to our health.

The raw restaurants in Brooklyn made the diet a little more exciting because I was able to have "lasagna, pizza, cheeseburgers, etc." Obviously, it wasn't lasagna made from flour, cheese and meat. "Raw" lasagna can use anything from flaxseed to spelt as the bread, raw cashew as the cheese, and mixed vegetables as the meat. It may not sound so delicious right now, but try eating salads and fruits for a week straight, then visiting a restaurant with foods that look similar to the unhealthy foods you're accustomed to eating. You'll devour it!

It's amazing how your taste buds along with your mental state change, allowing you to appreciate these foods in their natural state. A friend of mine named Howard actually accompanied me to a raw restaurant named "Raw Star" and decided to have the pizza. After eating the pizza, we stepped outside and he immediately started vomiting. At the time, I didn't understand why. Gaining knowledge about food and the human body over the years, I now understand that his body was not accustomed to having whole, unprocessed, natural foods. He had a diet primarily of flesh and fast food, so the raw food didn't agree with his body.

Some people like to say, "My body doesn't agree with the food," but on the contrary, it's not the food as one would believe; it's your body. This is one of the benefits of fasting; it prepares your body for a change in diet. Foods provided by nature are natural and in a healthy body, the food would not cause a reaction.

How we combine our foods on a daily basis can also cause reactions that disrupt the body. Gas, bloating, stomach cramping or infrequent stool elimination could be caused by how we are combining the food on our plate. There are some food combinations the human body has an easier time digesting. Next, we'll move into something that's even easier than fasting, a juice diet, or a raw food diet – food combining.

---

16. Marsden, Kathryn. *THE COMPLETE BOOK OF Food Combining*, First published in Great Britain in 2000 by Piakus, pg. 249

4

I GOT MAD GAS

FOOD COMBINING

The concept of food combining was introduced to me in 2016, while I researched easier ways to live a healthy lifestyle that don't involve completely eliminating all of the foods we enjoy daily. In practical terms, certain foods do not digest well together and others should be eaten on their own. This can alleviate digestive issues.

Fruits are packed with essential vitamins, minerals also known as antioxidants and should be eaten alone. **Antioxidants are extremely important because they protect our body from free radicals which damage our cells and cause cancer and other diseases.** Neuromelanin is a potent antioxidant when natural whole foods are consumed such as blueberries and blackberries. Before we continue to discuss food combining, I want to give a practical example of what happens to our body when free radicals begin to take over.

The human body is comprised of trillions of cells held together by electronic bonds. Cells are made of water, lipids, proteins, carbohydrates and nucleic acid. Within the center of the cell is DNA and RNA, which are also molecules that carry genetic information. I am ignoring certain structures of the molecules because it's quite complex and we don't need it here.

As oxygen makes its way through our body, it goes through a process called oxidation. Oxidation just means to break down. In our cells, there are couples that are called electrons that have bonds throughout our body.

Let's say we have ten couples that are running strong, but then one couple begins to have issues and the partner decides to cheat. The other partner now becomes a free radical, "damaged" and decides to leave the relationship (chemical bond). Instead of the damaged partner staying single for a while and practicing self-love, it becomes highly reactive and goes on to attach itself to a normal healthy couple in an attempt to replace their missing partner (electron), now damaging that couple. That group of damaged people latches itself on to another pair of healthy surrounding cells. The chain reaction continues resulting in the disruption of millions of nearby molecules.

Factors that cause oxidation, damage/breakdown to our cells and premature aging are:

- Poor diet

- Drugs and alcohol

- Cigarette/ marijuana smoke

- Radiation

- Stress/lack of sleep

- Aging

- Pollution

- Infection

Oxidation can be seen in a fruit that is exposed to air for a long period of time or rusting metal. Think about when you cut open an avocado or apple and it starts turning brown within minutes. Imagine this happening inside of your body. To prevent or reverse this destructive process, our bodies need a replenishment of antioxidant (anti-oxidation) molecules which we can get from vitamins and minerals found in natural foods.

Remember those natural foods that contain pigment we addressed earlier? That's what we're talking about, pigmented foods to resupply the melanin which is a powerful free radical scavenger. Melanin dominant people are free radical destroyers. A few fruits and veggies high in antioxidants are: cherries, red raspberries, grapes, wild blueberries, and the leader of the pack, Acai berries. (A list of supplements will be in my food shopping list.)

Hope you enjoyed that quick lesson, now back to food combining. Aside from the nutritious content, fruits have a high water content that assists with flushing toxins out and hydrating the body. "Fruit acids inhibit protein digestion because they restrict the production of stomach acids as well as destroying the protein-splitting enzyme, pepsin." [17]

Fruits combined with proteins or even starches prevent smooth digestion of all three foods and they can even remain in the stomach to rot. This can lead to gas, indigestion, heartburn, and bloating. Fruits are loners; they don't like company and would like easy transit through the digestive system without any interruption from chicken and rice. Once the fruits have entered the stomach, they go through the duodenum then into the small intestine to have all the vitamins and minerals absorbed.

On average, fruits take approximately thirty minutes to digest; so wait thirty minutes after eating fruits to consume protein, fats and carbs.

Remember, improper food combining is one of the leading causes of excess weight gain, skin eruptions, allergies, clogged veins and arteries, gas and colds; and the energy your body has to exert to break down and eliminate foods that don't go well together stresses your digestive system. "Eat fruit on an empty stomach. Either between meals or at the beginning of a meal, not with it, in the middle of it or immediately afterwards."[18]

Sidebar… I want to throw in a quick tip that also helps with digestion.

WHAT IS OIL PULLING?

Oil pulling gives a wakeup call to your digestive system to get ready to start processing food. It kills bacteria and triggers your body to start producing digestive enzymes. It is also known for reducing the bacteria on your teeth known as plaque. So, how do you oil pull? Take one tablespoon of extra-virgin coconut or sesame oil and swish it around your mouth for ten to fifteen minutes. Don't swallow any of the oil; spit it into the garbage when you're done. In the morning after you wake up and have a nice room temperature glass of water, you can oil pull next. Give it a try! I know it seems time consuming, but what isn't?

OXTAIL WITH RICE & PEAS

In my research, I learned some heart wrenching information about food combining. The last thing I would have ever expected was that proteins and starches don't digest well together in our bodies.

Proteins are: eggs, chicken, meat, pork, fish and lamb

Carbohydrates are: rice, pasta, potatoes, bread, quinoa, and oatmeal

As a woman from the Caribbean island of Jamaica, this truly broke my heart, because what is jerk, stew, curry chicken or oxtail without rice and peas?

There is a logical reason proteins and carbs don't want to be in a relationship together on your plate. They need different environments to be properly digested. Proteins need an acidic environment and carbs need a more or less neutral/alkaline environment to be properly digested. When you eat chicken with rice your stomach produces more hydrochloric acid and pepsin to breakdown the meal. This bad food combining is the leading cause of heartburn and acid reflux. If we pair our proteins with leafy greens, or carbohydrates with leafy greens and legumes, our bodies would thank us. Unfortunately, our stomachs aren't the best multi-taskers and have no way of separating proteins from carbs and ultimately decompose in the stomach.

What does all this mean? We have to do the work ourselves and eat these foods at different times. I did proper food combining for a few months and found the following to be true – less gas, bloating and overall digestive issues following each meal. I also noticed a slimming down of the waist. Food combining does a great job of reducing inflammation. **When we are internally inflamed, more calories are stored as fat which leads to weight gain.**

Proper food combining increases the amount of energy you can get from your foods because your stomach isn't producing an imbalanced secretion of alkaline and acid enzymes that overwork the gastrointestinal tract. This ultimately means we are getting more nutrients from our food because we have provided a stable environment for them to be assimilated.

The overall goal here is to give you options to change your diet, so you can have better health and longevity for yourselves, family and the community. If fasting, juicing or a raw food diet is too much for you now, even though I believe you all are very strong, food combining is a slower way of cleansing, but still a great option. Just minimize or eliminate your chicken, red meat, or lamb intake. They take a much longer time to digest than any other food processed through our bodies. I don't have pork on this list because it's a filthy animal filled with parasites that does not need to be consumed at all! Animal protein consumed on an empty stomach takes at least 5 hours to be processed. If it is mixed with starches it can take twice that amount of time or more.

Meats staying in the system for hours on end can cause them to rot in your gut, causing digestive issues. Your typical bacon (pig ass), eggs (chicken fetus), cheese (mucus) accompanied with a glass of milk (pus) is the worst possible breakfast you can have. We have to eat more foods that are biologically designed for our bodies.

My breakfast is not typical "breakfast foods" because breakfast just means you're breaking your fast from all the hours you just slept. If you enjoy Western breakfast foods, opt for organic oatmeal, buckwheat pancakes, or free-range organic eggs. Limit eggs to two times a week if still transitioning off dairy, especially if you have high blood pressure.

I don't claim to be vegan, vegetarian or pescatarian. In the near future I do plan to become vegan. At the moment I do everything in moderation to maintain balance along with seasonal cleanses. I abstain from pork. I eat red meat anywhere from two to four times a year if it's worth it. I have chicken up to two times a month and fish weekly. There is no need to eat animal protein in every meal you consume. My diet is high in dark leafy greens, vegetables, and a variety of nuts and beans. There are periods throughout the year when I go completely raw vegan for a month or more.

Ladies and gentlemen, I understand that eating healthy/organic can become costly, but there are markets like Trader Joes that have healthy food at an affordable cost. You have to live in this body for the rest of your life. Instead of allowing it to deteriorate due to a careless lifestyle, please take care of yourselves. Don't leave it to your husbands, wives, parents or children to have to feed, clothe or bathe you at an early age. Let's re-prioritize where our money goes, because one thing I don't want to see any more from my people is Gucci shoes and Chinese food!

Use this quick reference to food combine along with chart below. You can alternate the proteins and vegetables with the food shopping list in chapter fifteen. This is only an example.

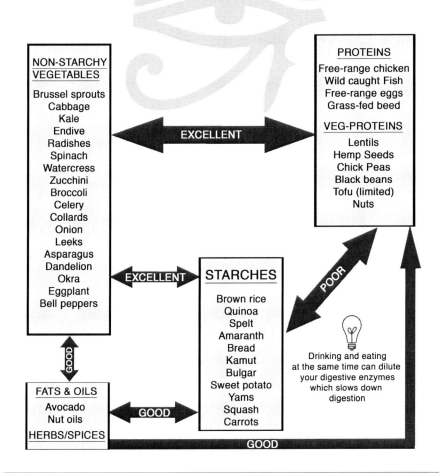

FOOD COMBINING CHART

NON-STARCHY VEGETABLES
Brussel sprouts
Cabbage
Kale
Endive
Radishes
Spinach
Watercress
Zucchini
Broccoli
Celery
Collards
Onion
Leeks
Asparagus
Dandelion
Okra
Eggplant
Bell peppers

PROTEINS
Free-range chicken
Wild caught Fish
Free-range eggs
Grass-fed beed

VEG-PROTEINS
Lentils
Hemp Seeds
Chick Peas
Black beans
Tofu (limited)
Nuts

EXCELLENT

EXCELLENT

STARCHES
Brown rice
Quinoa
Spelt
Amaranth
Bread
Kamut
Bulgar
Sweet potato
Yams
Squash
Carrots

POOR

GOOD

Drinking and eating at the same time can dilute your digestive enzymes which slows down digestion

FATS & OILS
Avocado
Nut oils
HERBS/SPICES

GOOD

GOOD

Fresh fruits are best eaten separately from other foods on an empty stomach. Eat melons on their own

Food Combining Day Example 1:

Breakfast (at 11am or 12pm)

- Have a bowl of fresh organic blueberries, strawberries, and blackberries.

- Wait at least twenty minutes to allow fruits to digest before enjoying your actual meal.

- Wild caught salmon (or black bean patty for vegans) with a salad. Salad can have kale, arugula, walnuts, dandelion, watercress, and two diced dates (for natural sweetness). Dates look like huge raisins but they are fruits that grow on trees called date palms. There are different kinds of dates, but I'm a fan of Medjool. They are naturally sweet, so if you have a dark leafy salad with diced up dates in it, you will love the flavor they give.

- Dressing: Extra virgin olive oil, lemon (if needed add a sprinkle of Himalayan sea salt if your taste buds don't like the olive oil and lemon by themselves).

Lunch (at 3pm)

- Quinoa with diced baked yams, steamed (or roasted) brussels sprouts and lentils.

To make brussels sprouts tasty, dice ten of them in half, put them in a large bowl; add 1 tablespoon of olive oil with paprika, thyme, and dried oregano. Preheat the oven to 375. Spread brussels sprouts on a baking sheet (not aluminum) paper baking sheet or glass. Roast for fifteen minutes.

When finished, sprinkle pink Himalayan sea salt on the brussels sprouts until you can ween off of using salt every meal. **Avoid seasoning foods with salt prior to them being finished cooking**. The salt tends to be absorbed and you end up adding more before you eat. Any cooked foods in aluminum containers deactivate the digestive juices; this can produce indigestion, acidosis (overproduction of acid that builds up in the blood, and ulcers).

Dinner (at 7pm)

- Dark green, leafy salad similar to the one made for "breakfast."

Food Combining Day Example 2:

Breakfast (at 12pm)

- Break your fast with a fresh bowl of organic fruits (oranges, grapefruits, or other citrus fruits go well together).

- Allow twenty to thirty minutes for digestion.

- Enjoy a bowl of organic oatmeal sweetened with a little date syrup or agave (can be found on Amazon.com). I choose date syrup because it is a natural sweetener and doesn't cause an acidic or inflammatory environment in your system.

Artificial sweeteners/syrups are poisonous to our bodies. Aunt Jemima was a slave who didn't know better so dump that syrup in the trash. Date syrup has vitamins, minerals, antioxidants, and amino acids. There's an ongoing controversy about some farmers using formaldehyde in the maple tree to keep the holes from closing so the sap can flow continuously. Formaldehyde is a known carcinogen that irritates and damages the body. It is also used in embalming deceased people.

Lunch (at 3:45pm)

- Organic, free-range chicken (for meat eaters) with a spinach, arugula, avocado, walnuts (soak in filtered water overnight for better digestion), and watercress salad

- Dressing: Balsamic vinaigrette

Dinner (at 7:00pm)

- Baked yams with chickpeas, brussels sprouts, quinoa, and stewed black beans.

To make quinoa, bring 1¼ cup of water or vegetable broth to a boil. Add ½ a cup of quinoa, turn heat on low, and cook for approximately 25 minutes. If you like your grains softer, you may need to cook for an additional 10 minutes. Quinoa can be prepared the same way as rice. You can add onion, thyme, and scallion to the water for more flavor. I also cook my quinoa or amaranth in homemade coconut milk.

Coconut milk from scratch: Add 1 cup of shredded coconut to 2.5 cups of filtered water and add to blender. Blend for 1-2 minutes. Strain or use a nut milk bag to drain milk.

Quick Tips:

Do not drink and eat at the same time. The fluid interferes with the body's natural ability to produce digestive enzymes, disrupting proper digestion. This is especially important when you're going to the beach or plan to be shirtless. Prevent bloating by consuming liquids 1 hour before or after the meal. This all just means a flat stomach.

Do not start your day with coffee. Start it with water to hydrate your digestive tract; coffee depletes the body of serotonin (the happy hormone). Coffee makes your kidneys work harder than they need to.

A few things to have at home to maximize gut health:

- Blueberries

- Coconut oil (one tablespoon daily) Heals and soothes inflamed tissues along the digestive tract. Improves nutrient absorption and combats parasites/bacteria.

- Turmeric and Ginger

- Pau d' Arco, licorice, and chai tea

---

17. Marsden, Kathryn. THE COMPLETE BOOK OF food combining, First published in Great Britain in 2000 by Piakus, pg. 26

18. Marsden, Kathryn. THE COMPLETE BOOK OF food combining. First published in Great Britain in 2000 by Piakus, pg. 27

5

DYING ON THE INSIDE

Some things won't make it into the colon from the top down, so if you have an ineffective digestive system, you have to start from the bottom and work your way up. I know you don't want to hear this, but colonics or even a warm water (filtered)/coffee enema is very beneficial to do at home. No one will even know! Enemas help with constipation, eliminate toxins, help clean out the colon, soften your poop, and detox the liver.

I do a Colonic Program once a year. It is something I have never seen offered at any other establishment. My holistic physician, Aisilda, has me abstain from food for one week. Yes, one week! In that week, I drink bentonite clay, psyllium husk and take vitamins only. Bentonite clay + Psyllium Husk assist with latching on to the poisons/toxins/fecal matter/prescription drugs that are lying trapped in your intestinal tract. The clay has an absorbent quality and the husk has a slippery lubricant quality that allows the filth to slide down to the intestinal tract.

Every day for seven days, I go to her office for a colonic. The purpose of not eating is to not add any additional food into my intestinal tract and to remove the matter sitting there. Let me explain something to you – the things I saw come out of my body almost made me pass out!

She catches everything I pass during the colonic into a bowl with a mesh spread out on the top. I saw dead parasites (worm-looking), masses of mucus, weird balls. She showed me prescription drugs I took five years ago because that was the last time I ever took medication, when I was pregnant with my daughter. Just pounds and pounds of waste. I lost ten pounds that week, mostly from my mid-section; but it's interesting because my midsection is small. You have to remember how the intestines are packaged so nicely in your middle area like a maze, so even the skinniest person will have pounds of waste in them.

I will tell you about two men who performed colonics and had great results! I monitored my brother, Safaree, while he did a five-day, green juice cleanse. He had approximately four to six fresh juices a day with water in between. His mind did begin to play tricks on him and there was a point where I thought he would attack me if I didn't feed him solid foods. After the juice diet was over, I accompanied him to get his first colonic ever.

This man had so much energy and strength when he was finished and completely changed his diet. This was a one-day colonic, but combined with his juice diet, he shredded the hell out of his midsection while eliminating pounds of waste!

My brother from another mother, Reggie Gray, performed the same seven-day colonic program that I did. I salute that man because he loves food. He became aware that it was time to do something about how he was looking, but more importantly, how he was feeling. Reggie was able to lose seventeen pounds in one week! This was all hidden in his stomach. I don't want to gross you out, so I won't attach pictures of what came out of us, along with our other friends that did it. A knife and fork can be dangerous weapons if we don't learn how to eat. If you do want to see pictures, you can reach me on **social media @neequa_09**.

6

GUCCI SHOES AND CHINESE FOOD

"One third of what you eat keeps you alive. The other three-quarters keeps your doctor alive."

−ANCIENT EGYPTIAN PROVERB

Our ancient ancestors knew that if you ate more than what is actually required for your body, several complications would arise – obesity, heart disease, diabetes, cancer and a host of other ailments associated with over-eating and improper elimination of these foods by our bodies; hence the above quote.

One thing I noticed a lot in my community was the overeating/poor eating habits of my brothers and sisters and the high-end clothing they wore. What good is having $1000 shoes, $500 belt/bag and $300 jeans if you feel like shit internally wearing them? So many people of color I know walk around with aches, joint pain, high blood pressure, diabetes, muffin top, constant headaches, asthma, and bad breath, but will have no problem cashing out at the most racist retail establishments such as Gucci. This is absolutely absurd to me and I hope it will soon be to you.

SAY NO TO CHINESE FOOD!

We cannot continue to patronize these filthy Chinese restaurants that cook almost all their food in old grease. The foods they are serving in our communities are not traditional Chinese food. What does this mean? They're not eating the garbage they're serving you.

I have been to Hong Kong and not once did I see General Tso Chicken. Think about the preparation of this mystery meat. It is deep fried in dark oil that is seldom changed, then smothered in good ol' diabetes sweet sauce. Congrats! You have now consumed a daily intake of 1500 or more calories in one meal.

To that I will add Lo Mein. The only kind of noodles I will treat myself to from time to time is the Guyanese version called Chow Mein. Chinese Lo Mein is packed with more sodium than you need in a single day! These refined carbs spike your sugar levels and will cost you about $6.50 and 1400 calories. Unstable blood sugar levels can cause food cravings, weakness, and lightheadedness. Then to top off these meals, we add oily egg rolls. Fried dough with "vegetables" if you could even still call them that after they have been smoldered by that old, hot grease. And don't forget your dipping sauce! The main culprit in that dipping sauce that keeps you running back for that glazed mystery meat and white rice is MSG.

"A long-term study carried out at the Harvard School of Public Health on 18,555 healthy women trying to get pregnant found that, for every 2% increase in the amount of calories a woman got from transfats, her risk of infertility increased by 73%.[19]

I want to summarize Dr. Jewel Pookrum's reason why people of color are more obese than any other race. "Melanin loves fat; the fat from these foods bonds to the melanin molecule and is used very slowly, sometimes recycled. We do not have to consume high fat diets to maintain our body fat. Melanin bodies already store fat because it binds with it; that is why we have so many overweight or obese people of color. Our bodies are structured differently physiologically."[20] She is not referring to natural fats such as avocados, this is about animal fat and fried greasy unnatural foods.

Again, race is not only skin deep. There is a disproportionate rise in obesity among people of color and a huge part of the reason that has been discovered by our black medical community is the melanin's ability to bind to fat in black/brown people.

Dr. Pookrum also tells us that our creator gave us this ability to store fat because we were originally living near the equator where most of the foods had very little fat. If it's 110 degrees every day; sugar, fat and protein, when broken down by the body give off energy. People of color can tolerate an enormous amount of heat when we eat properly and stay hydrated. This is because melanin has the capacity to absorb heat and dissipate it so you don't get hot.

We are sun people. If the melanin is functioning properly (you haven't put a pork chop in your mouth to cause the melanin to overheat) you should do just fine in a hot climate. Technically, we do not need air conditioners.

MSG

MSG is monosodium glutamine which basically is a flavor enhancer commonly added to Chinese food, processed meats, canned foods and soups. It is recognized as "safe" by the FDA (Food and Drug Administration). Before you get excited about the FDA deeming this additive safe, please understand that this is a government organization that does not have the best interest of the public at hand.

"The whole fakery in American research is almost entirely due to the pressures of the Rockefeller Medical Monopoly and the drug firms under their control, who routinely present elaborated faked "tests" to the Food and Drug Administration to obtain approval for new products, concealing harmful side effects, which often include liver and kidney damage, or death."[21]

Do you feel safe? I didn't think so. It's so interesting because while writing this book, I just happen to be working right in front of Memorial Sloan Kettering Cancer Center located on East 61st street and York Avenue in Manhattan. Why do I bring this up, you might ask? "Virtually all of the chemotherapeutic agents now approved by the FDA for use or testing in human cancer patients are highly toxic to markedly immuno-suppressive and highly carcinogenic in rats and mice, themselves producing cancers in a wide variety of body organs."[22]

Understand that disease is a multi-billion dollar business, all relatively run by the same organizations. If you don't voluntarily make time to upkeep your health, you will have to involuntarily make time to reverse your dis-ease. Processed food, tap water, synthetic drugs (prescription), and sitting on your ass all day are decreasing the production of melanin.

Now, where was I? Yes, MSG. Studies have shown that there are harmful effects of MSG such as anxiety, bloating, headache, eczema, muscle tightness, heart palpitations, asthma attacks, and increased blood pressure. People of color tend to be more sensitive to MSG due to the melanin in our bodies which we discussed earlier in the book.

Chinese people are infamous for making imitation everything, down to the food. When I was in Hong Kong, I was warned of foods to stay away from because they were fake. A few things to stay clear of were chemically created eggs, beef which is actually pork (done with beef extract, powder and caramel), green peas, honey, walnuts (inside the walnut were concrete chips and paper), and the infamous plastic rice made from potatoes and plastic. WTF!

So, here's the thing, I don't expect everyone to read this and become vegans, vegetarians or any of the "ans" right away. I want you to be aware of what you are putting inside of your body as opposed to outside of your body. I want you to feed your body Gucci if that makes sense.

GUCCI ON THE INSIDE

Don't get me wrong. Our ancient African ancestors dressed fly, but it was for spiritual and curative purposes. They definitely took pride in hygiene, what they wore, and they most definitely had the iced-out jewels on that represented higher consciousness. But their first concern was what they were putting inside their bodies because they knew unwholesome foods would obstruct their path on becoming their higher self; becoming God on Earth.

The reason I started with fasting/cleansing options before supplements is because there are various situations in which taking vitamins isn't doing anything for your body because it's too toxic to absorb the nutrients. "In a body full of wastes and poisons, it is impossible for them to enter into your blood stream in a clean state and become "efficiency-giving" vital substances."[23]

When detoxification of the eliminatory systems occurs, especially the colon and liver, the body has improved its ability to absorb nutrients from foods and supplements. Before listing vitamins and herbs essential for the vitality of people of color, I want to take time to share the final resort to a change in diet through slow transitioning.

"SLOW MOTION FOR ME"

There are some of us who may have our priorities in order, but still don't feel we can afford whole nutritious foods. I believe you can because once you follow this plan, you'll be eating less because the food will be sustained in your body longer. Instead of buying or eating three to five times a day, you would eat two to three times, allowing for you to now invest in quality foods.

Whole foods keep you fuller longer because of all the nutrients provided. Instead of eating from 7:00am to 10:00pm, you will eat from 11am-7pm – eight hours of eating followed by sixteen hours of fasting. This has been called "intermittent fasting," but our ancestors have been practicing this for donkey years, because they knew overeating shortens your lifespan. What sense is it to be over-fed and under nourished?

Of course, you will see people in your lifetime that broke all the rules of nutrition and ate meat, rice, sugar, candy, drank liquor, smoked cigarettes, weed, and maybe even dabbled in a little coke; who knows? I know people like that who lived until their mid-nineties, but they were nowhere near being the poster child for good health. They were completely dependent on the help of others and lived in complete discomfort for half of their life. Length of life has nothing to do with quality of life. The medical monopoly wants to make you comfortable living with disease not, curing it. The word "cure" is foreign in western medicine.

Shortening your time frame for eating will allow for proper digestion and elimination. It will also allow you to save more money because you won't be eating and snacking all day. Give yourself about two to three months to start seeing a difference in your body. You will get used to eating at these times and will no longer crave food as soon as you wake up.

The myth that you need to eat breakfast for energy has gone on for too long. The food you eat first thing in the morning is NOT what gives you energy. That food has to go through the stomach and intestines to be processed by the liver and pancreas before being distributed into your cells for energy. This can take anywhere from four to eight hours or longer depending on what you ate. If you are constipated, this so-called energy breakfast food can take days to be used for energy.

There are rare people, like my friend Keon, who can watch a video about the negative health effects of processed foods and become a vegan the next day. I know that it isn't the easiest thing to transition, so taking it slow is better than not taking any direction towards better health at all. Here is a short example of how to slowly transition:

White rice > Brown rice > Wild rice > Quinoa > Kamut > Spelt

White sugar > Honey > Date sugar > Agave > Stevia

White Flour > Wheat Flour > Sprouted grains > Coconut/Almond flour > Spelt flour

Pork > Red meat > Chicken > Turkey > Fish > No animal products

Cow's milk > Almond milk > Pea milk > Hemp milk

Table salt > Sea salt > Pink Himalayan sea salt > No salt

Fried > Boiled > Roasted > Baked > Lightly steamed

Iceberg lettuce > Romaine lettuce > Kale > Arugula > Watercress

Corn oil > Olive oil > Coconut oil > Hempseed oil > Grapeseed oil > Avocado oil

The goal is to get your digestive system moving at a normal rate. The medical industry tells you three movements a day or three a week are normal. Let's do some math here, you eat three meals a day for seven days. That's twenty-one meals you have consumed. Let's say you took a dump four times for the week because you got lucky. Where are the other seventeen meals? I'll let you figure that out.

19. Dr. Jewel Pookrum. Published March 24, 2016. "Differences between Africans and other races and cell regeneration." https://youtu.be/yJIF6BYS9po

20. Gerson, Charlotte and Bishop, Beata Eustace. *Healing The Gerson Way,* (2013), pg. 39.

21. Mullins, Eustace. *MURDER BY INJECTION*; The Story of the Medical Conspiracy Against America, (1995), pg. 97.

22. Mullins, Eustace. *MURDER BY INJECTION*; The Story of the Medical Conspiracy Against America, (1995), pg. 108.

23. Ehret, Arnold, Annotated, Revised, and Edited by Prof. Spira Prof. Arnold Ehret's. *Mucusless Diet Healing System* Revised, (November 2015), pg.48

7

FOR THE LOVE OF HENNESSEY

"Lemme Get a Henny and Red Bull"

-RAYMOND A MUSCAT

Typically, in neighborhoods of color, you're able to find a liquor store on almost every corner. As I said earlier, this is no coincidence since well over a majority of them are not owned by any people of color; just like most of the businesses in the inner cities are not black owned. As a black woman having grown up around so many amazing men of color, I can clearly see how easy it is to fall victim to alcoholism or excessive alcohol drinking.

- One in three black men can expect to go to prison in their lifetime.

- Black and brown men are three times more likely to be searched during a traffic stop than white men.

- African Americans were twice as likely to be arrested and almost four times as likely to experience the use of force during encounters with police.

- Black/Brown males are incarcerated at a rate six times higher than white males.

- Students of color face harsher punishments in school than their white peers.

- Once convicted, men of color receive longer sentences compared to white offenders.

- Wages grow at a 21% slower rate for black former inmates compared to white ex-cons.

- 45% of black men are in prison.

- 17.5% of the unemployed are black men.

- 36% of black men are alcoholics. [23]

What does all of this mean? In America, people of color are stressed the f&%# out! Despite these alarming and shocking stats, you all must take responsibility now more than ever before and learn to heal yourselves.

I will summarize Dr. Frances Cress Welsing view on the system in place here. We have been victimized by a system that doesn't want us to be strong and functional. The system is not broken, the system is working perfectly because it was never meant to work for you. If your plan is to live here in America, where there is still plenty of opportunity despite racism then it is time to fight back. Fight back by saying I will not allow this system to genocide me.[24]

If anyone needs to value and respect themselves, it is black and brown men and women. People with no melanin are a very small percentage of the global population and the only way for them to exist was to enslave non-whites, and divide and conquer entire countries based on their differences, while holding true to their own similarities.

How did they do this? In short, they organized a ruthless, savage military force behind their goal and executed their mission seamlessly. Their main objective was to ensure their survival. Don't forget about the free labor from your ancestors to finance the Industrial Revolution during the 18th century. These inventions permanently changed society and what did people of color get for it? Nothing. What will we get in the future? Nothing, if we don't work towards what every other race has – UNITY. Not depending on a new puppet president who uses our struggles as a campaign ploy and forgets about us once elected. We need each other to elevate.

I understand that taking steps to bettering yourself can be quite challenging. For that reason, I suggest taking baby steps towards our ultimate goal of cleansing our bodies and being free of dis-ease – allowing us think. "A black person's level of thinking (mental growth) needed to solve their race's problems cannot be achieved with a low amount of melanin caused by an under-stimulated pineal gland." [25]

The pineal gland secretes melanin and stimulates the brain, spinal cord, sensory organs; everything associated with the nervous system. Therefore, the function of the brain is reduced even more following bad diets, excessive drug use, and alcohol intake.

Dear Owner,
Please Stop Drinking
Love, Your Liver

The reduction of alcohol intake will allow your liver to function at optimal levels. Your liver is the second largest organ in the body and has a lot of responsibility in eliminating toxins just like the colon. The digestive system transports synthetic chemicals (prescription drugs, pesticide residue) into the liver, which keeps the bloodstream clear of anything it deems poisonous to the body. All your body's blood flows through the liver for processing and purification.

Since the liver has a full-time job already with not many lunch breaks, it goes into overload and becomes exhausted. Every sixty seconds this amazing organ filters, cleans and recycles roughly one liter of blood. Bile is a fluid secreted by the liver to aid in digestion of cholesterol and fats from the intestines. The liver's ability to produce bile is much more effective with melanin.

Your gallbladder is under your liver and stores the incoming bile. When we eat fats and proteins, the gallbladder is triggered to squeeze itself empty like a sponge after approximately twenty minutes. The stored bile then travels down the common bile duct into the intestines. A lot of people have a bile tube that is filled with gallstones. If these gallstones grow, they can cause intense pressure on the liver, causing less bile production.

When you're in the club "making it rain" and popping bottles, your poor liver is praying for dear life! When that Henny's in the system, it produces a toxic enzyme called acetaldehyde, which can damage liver cells and cause permanent scarring. Don't forget the harm it does to the melanin producing brain and stomach lining. Alcohol acts as a diuretic (increases the release of urine) which ultimately dehydrates you and forces the liver to find water from other sources. The severe dehydration is part of the reason why, after "turning-up," you wake-up with a pounding headache.

Over time, heavy drinking can then lead to alcoholic liver disease. If you're the type of person that has no self-control once you're out, it's time to minimize the partying. The benefit is, your liver will thank you and you won't get any text messages from your boyfriend or girlfriend trying to ruin your night out.

Nourish your liver by combining herbs like milk thistle, comfrey, and dandelion. You will find more herbs after the shopping list section in this book.

LATE NIGHT EATING

After you leave the club, you're hungry from all that drinking, so you stuff your face at a fast food restaurant and go to sleep. This is one of the worst things you can do. Late night eating fills up the digestive system. While your body is trying to get rest, your digestive system would like to join in and rest too. Late night eating and sleeping can cause heartburn. Food gets stuck in the small intestine because you're in a reclined position.

Your intestine will have a hard time pushing food through in a reclined position, and this causes the food to get trapped and rot. Your body is just not at peak efficiency to break foods down, so this can speed up the aging process.

There is a time frame I like to call "magic sleep healing," when your body is going through cell regeneration and detoxification. This is the time when your glands are functioning at their best. Melatonin and melanin are being secreted through the pineal gland and go throughout the body. That time is from approximatly 10:00pm to 3:00am and the room should be in complete darkness. The body cannot perform this function optimally if it is still digesting foods throughout the night.

Eating at night is just as bad as eating as soon as you wake up. All that magic sleep healing goes right out the window the moment you wake up and have a cup of coffee with bacon, egg, and cheese on a roll. You need to start your morning with warm water and lemon to activate your digestive system properly and flush out all the mucus and toxins your body has accumulated overnight. Water helps dissolve and remove materials from within that we do not want in our body.

HOW TO DO #2

Over time, excessive late night eating along with eating wrong foods will cause constipation. Over sixty million people in the United States are constipated with over five million prescriptions written out yearly for laxatives. To make matters worse, we aren't even sitting on the toilet properly. Yes, there is a proper way to do number two, which you will see in the sketch below.

PPP
Proper Poop Position

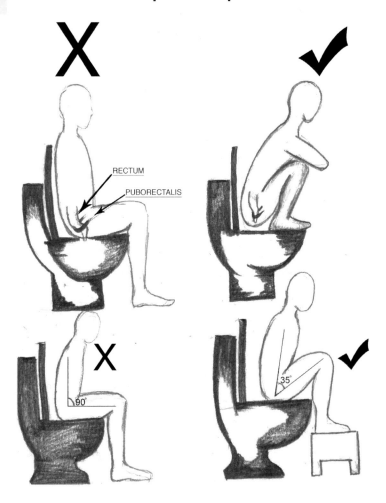

The modern toilet (Westernized) is causing constipation. Sitting in the commonly practiced ninety degree position, the passage of your intestines are disrupted and sealed off. This usually leads people to strain during a bowel movement because their bodies aren't in a squatting position.

Your knees must be higher than your hips to have a proper bowel movement. The normal thirty-five degree position allows the natural flow of poop to exit your rectum. The average time to drop a load in the squatted position is approximately fifty-one seconds, while the ninety degree way is 130 seconds respectively. This positon is normal in our ancestral culture.

When I visited Japan, I noticed all their toilets were half the height of the toilets in America. I know we aren't all going to go out and buy a new toilet, so a simple solution is to get a stool to rest your feet on so that your knees are above your hips. I use my daughter's step stool. No need to buy some overpriced object when you can use anything that will raise your knees.

In the diagram, you will see the puborectalis muscle, which is wrapped around the rectum. This muscle is like a sling, which contracts and relaxes to control the pooping process. It also pulls the rectum forward to create the anorectal (acute) angle between the anus and the rectum. Squatting widens the angle while relaxing and straightening the rectum to allow for less straining and a clear passage for stool to exit the anus.

The next time you're on your way to drop a load, follow these rules for an easy go. This will not eliminate all constipation issues if you still have a diet in high processed foods and refined sugars, because your poop will still be hard as a rock. Stop taking pills to solve your problems. "Let your food be your medicine and your medicine be your food."

YOU GOT A LIGHT?

I would also like to take a moment to address cigarette smoking. Cigarettes are full of high-grade carcinogens and toxic agents. Remember those free radicals we addressed earlier in the food combining section? There are over one hundred million of them in every pull you take. Have you ever noticed that heavy cigarette smokers look twice their age and have immense wrinkles? Nicotine deactivates melanin molecules and delays transmittal of signals from the skin to the brain.

I can usually spot a heavy smoker from a mile away because their melanin is discolored and unhealthy looking. If you are a heavy smoker, your melanin will become toxic and you will have much more brain fog/forgetfulness than non–smokers. **Melanin binds to toxic chemicals in hopes of ejecting them out of your body**. The more melanin you have, the more addicted you are to drugs and alcohol due to the bonding feature of this molecule. This is why we have a higher rate of dis-ease, especially cancer. Cancer is a proliferation of degenerate cell colonies in the organism that migrate throughout the body seeking shelter. While seeking shelter, they are robbing the healthy cells of their nutrients. "Cancer is a disease of nutrition."

"The chemotherapy drugs include alkylating agents which actually inhibit cell growth… Sloan Kettering also bypasses the possibility of stimulating the immune system to respond to cancer growth, which is the normal method the body uses to fight disease."[26] If you still plan to live a careless lifestyle because you trust in the medical monopoly, here is another fun fact…

"Not only do the boards of Memorial Sloan Kettering have direct ties to the Rockefellers; they are also closely linked with defense industries, the CIA, and chemical drug firms. It is no accident that they serve on the board of an institution whose recommendations on cancer treatment mean literally billions in profits to those who are in the right position to take advantage of them. And you thought this was a charitable organization! The fact is the Memorial Sloan Kettering and the American Cancer Society are the principal organizational functionaries, with the American Medical Association, of the Rockefeller Medical Monopoly."[27]

Now that you have done your fast/diet and your liver is squeaky clean, ready to carry out its daily work, we can introduce vitamins and herbs that would love to be absorbed by your alkaline blood.

24. Frances Cress. Published Aug. 26, 2017. The Cress Theory of Color Confrontation and Racism. https://youtu.be/7rzWf7Tn3ak

25. Afrika, Llaila. Melanin- What Makes Black People Black. Seaburn Publishing group, New York (2009), pg.12.

26. Mullins, Eustace. *MURDER BY INJECTION*; The Story of the Medical Conspiracy Against America, (1995), pg. 98.

27. Mullins, Eustace. *MURDER BY INJECTION*; The Story of the Medical Conspiracy Against America, (1995), pg. 76.

8

PILL POPPIN

To continue on this journey of health, I want to address essential vitamins for nourishment of our melanin and prolonged health. Melanin is brown to black in color and absorbs all kinds of energy including sunlight. Darker skin prevents sun damage and regulates conversion of cholesterol into vitamin D.

VITAMIN D

People of color need to spend a lot more time in the sun. Everybody has the ability to produce vitamin D when their skin is exposed to ultraviolet light. This light (sun) activates vitamin D in our body, which makes its way through the blood stream to the liver and kidneys. We need vitamin D to absorb and utilize calcium. But what about the people of color in the northern hemisphere during the winter months? They become extremely vitamin D deficient because our melanin blocks the ultraviolet rays.

That little bit of sun exposure in the winter months is not enough to pierce through that beautiful skin of yours in order to produce vitamin D on its own. We need approximately two hours of sun four times a week as opposed to less melanated men who just need fifteen minutes, three times a week.

Research has also shown that an overweight person's exposure to the sun doesn't produce the same amount of vitamin D as compared to someone of normal weight. Why? The vitamin D may be hiding in the fat cells. The darker the skin, the more difficult it is to produce vitamin D.

It has become increasingly apparent that vitamin D protects against chronic conditions such as cardiovascular disease, diabetes, and prostate cancer, all of which are more prevalent among men of color than whites. "More than 6000 black men die each year from prostate cancer."[28]

That's the word according to a new study conducted at Northwestern University Feinberg School of Medicine. In this study, 63% of African Americans were deficient in vitamin D compared to 18% of white men. "When vitamin D levels fall below 20ml/dl, the bone starts to become brittle in adults and in kids it causes rickets,"[29] noted Adam Murphy MD, an African-American physician. People of color need up to six times more exposure to the sun than whites. Vitamin D from supplements or natural sunlight prevents cancer of the prostate, breast, ovary, and brain.

The general recommendation for vitamin D supplementation is 600 IUs/day, but like I said, we are not the same. "The incidence of some 16 different types of cancer has been linked with vitamin D insufficiency… Dark skinned people living more than 30 degrees from the equator may find that they need vitamin D in diet or supplements all year round, since D deficiency may cause several of the problems of the dark-skinned living in areas with limited sun."[30] Vitamin D deficiency causes the body to pull calcium from the bones (including teeth) to restore the bloods pH balance.

A final note on the sun that I found so interesting is the sun itself does not cause skin cancer, rather it's the conditions of the person in the sun that can cause skin cancer. In essence, if the person in the sun consumes too many sugary products, processed foods, mucus forming dairy, the sun permeating the skin of that overly toxic person is what leads to skin cancer. The sun's rays create an acidic environment which causes these toxicities to rise to the surface, therefore becoming a cata- lyst (increasing the rate of a chemical reaction) causing the cancer. This is mainly an issue for those lacking melanin.

Over 90% of African-Americans may have vitamin D deficiency

Recommended amount for Melanated people: 5000 IU a day. Must be taken with calcium and magnesium (see a holistic physician for verification). During spring and summer, supplementation is not necessary. Stand outdoors in sun for one to two hours a day.

Food sources of Vitamin D: Herring, fresh squeezed orange juice, halibut, trout, alfalfa, oatmeal, sweet potato, yam and salmon.

VITAMIN C

If there is one group lacking when it comes to vitamin C intake, it is people of color. Vitamin C is used up in large amounts when we are in a stressful situation, traumatized, injured, suffering mental or emo- tional stress, etc. Along with the high level of stress, black people have the added issues of exposure to inner city pollutants, smoking, and low-quality diet.

The adrenal glands, located right on top of the kidneys, are where vitamin C is most concentrated and is readily available if a stressful situation arises. For a man of color, that can happen almost any minute of the day, just walking down the street. Notably, men of color don't express their anger very well, if they express it at all. That anger is a powerful form of energy which usually is bottled up and can health problems. If you don't cope well with stress, vitamin C must be a staple in your cabinet. The mind influences the condition of the body.

This antioxidant is required for healthy gums, collagen growth (protein found in the skin), prevents cancer, reduces high blood pressure, fights heart disease, and protects your memory/thinking as you age.[1]

"Men who consume low levels of vitamin C are more likely to develop defective sperm than those consuming the recommended daily allowance of 60mg."[31]

Recommended amount: 1000-2000mg a day divided in doses if you're healthy. If you're sick, take up to 3,000mg. (The body absorbs more when it is sick).

Food sources of Vitamin C: Guavas, kale, kiwi fruit, broccoli, Brussel sprouts, lemons, papayas, strawberries, oranges, spinach, sweet potatoes, and mangoes

I prefer to get my vitamin C from whole plant and fruit sources. The reason is when looking for supplements I notice that almost all brands get their vitamin C from 100% ascorbic acid and L-ascorbic acid. This is not the same as vitamin C but is an isolated nutrient that is part of the vitamin. Moreover, ascorbic acid can be made by mixing corn syrup and hydrochloric acid rather than extracting it from natural foods. Most of us should know by now that this country typically takes the short inexpensive route when it comes to quality and sales. Vitamin C should have bioflavonoids, tyrosinase, ascorbinogen, and rutin.

CALCIUM/MAGNESIUM

Magnesium gets used up quite quickly every time the body produces stress hormones. Calcium is vital for strong teeth and bones. Calcium supplements can also help lower blood pressure, fight heart disease, and diabetes. Being that a majority of African Americans (75%) are lactose intolerant, that calcium must be retrieved through non-dairy products and supplements.

Our ancestors consumed very little dairy in their diets. Melanated people lack the enzyme necessary to break down dairy products. If you find yourself gassy, bloated, or running straight to the bathroom after consuming dairy products, you my friend, are lactose intolerant. The reason calcium and magnesium are paired together in this section is because they normally interact in the body. "Calcium and magnesium must be taken together to work their best, with roughly twice the amount of magnesium as calcium...Calcium supplements should not be taken by people suffering from kidney stones or kidney disease."[32]

Recommended amount: 1000mg of calcium and 2000mg of magnesium daily (plant-based)

Food sources of Calcium and Magnesium: salmon, kale, collard greens, dandelion greens, oats, spinach, broccoli; brown rice, figs, avocados, peaches, bananas and sesame seeds.

Note: Minerals best absorbed when linked to a source of protein.

ZINC

Zinc is so important for men of color, especially with the growing prevalence of prostate cancer. Zinc is essential in prostate gland function. Studies have shown that a lack of zinc in men can cause infertility and sperm issues. Zinc is well known for its immune building/

cold fighting capabilities. "Zinc lozenges have been found to reduce the duration of colds by more than 40 percent."[33] Zinc also grows and repairs body tissues.

Recommended amount: 25-50mg daily

Food sources: Chickpeas, lentils, cashews, quinoa, sweet potatoes, brown rice and oats.

Note: Minerals best absorbed when linked to a source of protein.

SELENIUM and VITAMIN E

These two supplements are especially important in people that smoke cigarettes or marijuana. Selenium has antioxidant properties that assist in preventing blood clots, which lead to stroke and heart attack. Vitamin E helps with blood circulation, repairing damaged tissue from poor diet, drinking, and smoking. These powerful antioxidants are essential for the body to function normally. Without them, you can suffer from muscle weakness, impaired eyesight, or being more susceptible to infections. They are known to help people with diabetes by boosting immune function. These supplements are best taken together as they facilitate each other's absorption.

Recommended amount: 400 to 800 IU of Vitamin E daily (unless you have an overactive thyroid or rheumatic heart disease; check with your physician first as you may require a lower dosage such as 200IU).

Selenium recommended amount: 200 micrograms a day (verify amount with a holistic or medical physician).

Food sources: Garlic, salmon, wheat germ, brown rice, Brazil nuts, sweet potatoes, walnuts, broccoli and onions.

VITAMIN A (BETA CAROTENE)

Prevents night blindness and other eye issues. It's an antioxidant that enhances immunity and protects the body from free radical damage.

Recommended amount: 10,000IU

Food Sources: Sweet potatoes, papayas, yellow squash, asparagus, kale, spirulina, cantaloupe, pumpkin, and watercress.

VITAMIN B COMPLEX
(Combination of B2, 5, 6, and 12)

Tones the gastrointestinal tract and prevents kidney stones while maintaining healthy skin, hair, liver, and nerves. B12 is great for red blood cell production and assists with carb, fat, and protein digestion. B5 plays a vital role in reducing inflammation in the body.

Recommended amount: 300mg

- **Food Sources:** Brown rice, broccoli, brussels sprouts, oatmeal, avocados, spinach and asparagus.

PROBIOTICS

Trillions of bacteria live in the large intestine. Most are harmless or actively help complete digestion by processing the left over nutrients that weren't able to be digested by the body's enzymes. However, some of these bacteria can cause disease. Dis-ease enters our body through the airways, digestive tract, penis, vagina, and the skin.

Probiotics are a blend of live, healthy bacteria that colonize your digestive system and promote proper digestion. An imbalance in the intestinal tract means there are too many bad bacteria and not enough good bacteria. Our intestinal tract can get loaded with yeast, fungus, and mold. Benefits of probiotics include minimizing bloating, gas, itating bowel movements, preventing constipation, and diarrhea.

Healthy probiotics live in our gastrointestinal tract, but du cooked foods, flesh foods, dairy, and antibiotics, they begin to die off leaving us defenseless against over production of yeast or other diseases. Fasting monthly and preparing our own foods can minimize bacteria consumption. Some probiotics prevent the absorption of dietary fat in the intestine. The fat is then excreted through the colon rather than stored in the body.

Recommended amount: 50 billion – 100 Billion CFU (colony forming units) in a capsule daily on an empty stomach (verify with a nutritionist how much is best for you).

DIGESTIVE ENZYMES

Enzymes improve the breakdown of protein, fat, and carbs and help us to utilize nutrients better. Since a lot of us are eating things that are not in their natural state, our bodies have a tough time breaking these things down with the natural enzymes created by our bodies. Enzymes provide some extra help that can be beneficial to our digestive system. They can also help split up partially digested dietary proteins.

GINSENG ROOT

Ginseng root (panax) is an antioxidant discovered over 5000 years ago, known to manage sexual dysfunction (erectile dysfunction) as well as lower blood sugar, boost energy, and reduce stress. It gives your immunes system an overall boost while enhancing brain function.

YOHIMBE

Bark from a tree in Central Africa used to treat erectile dysfunction. Increase sexual desire (not that any men need that!)

I don't want you to go out and buy everything on this list. Get a physical to see what vitamins you are low in. Also go based on how you are feeling. If you feel that you are a person that is highly stressed then get vitamin C supplement or increase your intake of foods containing vitamin C. Maybe you have low energy, supplement with some ginseng while changing your diet. Be your own judge. I personally prefer to get my vitamins and minerals in the foods I eat, but I do supplement from time to time.

We have to build our immune system so it is ready to defend us against bacteria, viruses, and anything unnatural to the body. I have not "caught" a cold in years. We don't catch colds, we create them by having a weak immune system. I work outside all year round and don't dress "properly" and the weather still does not affect whether I get sick or not, my dietary practices do.

28. Afua, Queen. *Sacred Woman; A Guide To Healing The Feminine Body, Mind, And Spirit*, Published by The Random House Publishing Group (2000), pg. 345

29. Reacher, James. Is Vitamin D Deficiency High Among African-American Men? September 20, 2011. https://prostate.net/articles/is-vitamin-d-deficiency-high-among-african-american-men

30. Kauffman, Joel M. *Malignant Medical Myths*, Infinity publishing (2006), pg.233.

31. Dr. Jewel Pookrum. Published March 24, 2016. *Differences between Africans and other races and cell regeneration.* https://youtu.be/yJIF6BYS9po

32, 33. Walker, Marcellus A. M.D and Singleton, Kenneth B., M.D. *Natural Health for African Americans*, New York, (February 1999), pg. 162-172.

9

"A WEH DI BLOODCLAAT DEM A TALK BOUT?"

-SAFAREE SAMUELS

Dis-ease means your body is losing the race against eliminating waste. At the most basic level, we are taught about these the different "systems" in the body and their functions in school. In holistic African centered science, we believe all disease is a blood disease. Our bodies are made up of the central nervous system, digestive system, urinary system, lymphatic system, muscular system, endocrine system, and reproductive system. What we are not taught properly is that these "systems" are family and are related to each other. These systems are blood relatives working together to live harmoniously. So look at the organs as a family unit from now on that have the same genetic makeup.

MELANIN BODY

Let's break down what makes a human in the simplest form possible. Atoms are made up of electrons, protons, and neutrons (all melanin particles) and they join together to form molecules. Water is a molecule made from hydrogen and oxygen atoms. More than 93% of the human body is made from just oxygen, carbon, and hydrogen. Most of the oxygen is combined with hydrogen to make water. We are roughly seventy percent water. This is the order of how the human body comes together by just a few chemical substances.

MOLECULES > CELLS > TISSUE > ORGANS > BODY SYSTEMS

Humans are made up of over 100 trillion cells. Cells doing the same thing get grouped together and make body tissues. There are four different types of tissues. A bunch of cells grouped together can make skin, heart muscle, fat, and even blood. Blood is tissue in liquid form. Another kind of tissue combines to make organs like the stomach. Then organs come together to make a "system."

BLOOD

"The magnitude and implication of apparent race differences in hemoglobin values, published in the American Journal of Clinical Nutrition, 1975 makes it clear that the differences in blood composition and content in various races is a genetic standard and to assume the variation is pathological when compared to another race's blood values and would ensue action nutritional and otherwise that may be **lethal to the racial group** assumed to be pathologic."[34]

Hemoglobin is one of the many elements that make up blood and is different according to race. Hemoglobin is the oxygen carrying protein in red blood cells. It carries oxygen into the blood and carbon dioxide out of the blood. Low levels of red blood cells means low levels of oxygen. Why is this important? Improper blood flow means your body can't get all the oxygen and nutrients it needs.

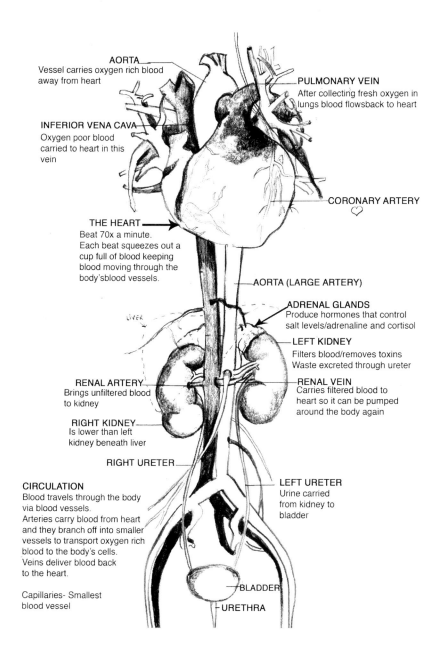

AORTA
Vessel carries oxygen rich blood away from heart

PULMONARY VEIN
After collecting fresh oxygen in lungs blood flowsback to heart

INFERIOR VENA CAVA
Oxygen poor blood carried to heart in this vein

CORONARY ARTERY

THE HEART
Beat 70x a minute.
Each beat squeezes out a cup full of blood keeping blood moving through the body'sblood vessels.

AORTA (LARGE ARTERY)

ADRENAL GLANDS
Produce hormones that control salt levels/adrenaline and cortisol

LIVER

LEFT KIDNEY
Filters blood/removes toxins Waste excreted through ureter

RENAL ARTERY
Brings unfiltered blood to kidney

RENAL VEIN
Carries filtered blood to heart so it can be pumped around the body again

RIGHT KIDNEY
Is lower than left kidney beneath liver

RIGHT URETER

CIRCULATION
Blood travels through the body via blood vessels.
Arteries carry blood from heart and they branch off into smaller vessels to transport oxygen rich blood to the body's cells.
Veins deliver blood back to the heart.

LEFT URETER
Urine carried from kidney to bladder

Capillaries- Smallest blood vessel

BLADDER

URETHRA

The circulatory system is similar to the underground subway system. The blood is the cars that carry food, oxygen, waste products, hormones, and other essentials from organ to organ. The heart is the train control center that drives the blood along the route. The blood vessels are the train tracks by which blood travels. "In poor blood circulation, the blood gets overloaded with waste (liquid manure) and becomes thick and slow to move."[35] Slightly acidic blood decreases the ability of cells, tissue and organs to get oxygen and nutrients. Poor blood circulation is one of the problems prevalent amongst people of color.

Main purposes of Blood:

- Carries nutrients, oxygen and water to the tissues (cells).

- Carries waste to the excretory organs to excrete them.

- Fights infections through white blood cells

- Provides materials from which glands make their hormones.

- Distributes heat evenly throughout the body to regulate body temperature.

- Stops hemorrhaging through clotting.

MELANIN AND HIGH BLOOD PRESSURE

The pressure exerted by the blood against the walls of arteries is called blood pressure. Your blood pressure reading has two numbers. The higher number on top measures the pressure when your heart contracts. The lower number measures the pressure when the heart is at rest. 120/80 is considered normal. When it is over 140/90, it's considered dangerous. Medical science has an interesting answer as to why high blood pressure is more common in black/Hispanic people of African descent. I've seen some medical articles that say it's because colored people have a higher risk of diabetes and are more overweight than other races. Thank you for that lack of information.

I found a few articles that seem like they are on to something, but don't get excited because the last thing they want is for you to know that you're different on the inside too. The most logical article stated that black/brown people "may have a gene that makes us more sensitive to salt." Duh! As I mentioned earlier, our blood is not the same as that of European people, but they base our bloodwork on the values of European people.

"Melanin-dominant body is programmed for vegetable consumption as a source of protein and minerals, not flesh. As more melanin-dominant people begin to digest flesh as a source of protein, mineral blockage diseases become a major problem."[36]

The human body has over a trillion cells. Every cell has an information center in the middle called a nucleus. This is the control center/brain of the cell. Melanin is a biochemical highly present in every organ in people of color. Melanin is produced in excess when there is weakness in the body to protect you. An undernourished pineal gland will hamper the production of melanin.

The brain of every cell has genetic material called DNA. You inherit DNA from your parents and it identifies who you are. As Dr. Laila O. Afrika teaches us, melanin is not just what makes us brown to black, it is chemical particles all throughout our bodies. "Melanin has a free radical behavior. It will attack harmful synthetic chemicals (i.e. preservatives, food additives, drugs, cocaine, crack, marijuana, Viagra, caffeine) and attach to them in attempt to transport them elsewhere or neutralize them."[37]

For this reason, the melanin and unnatural chemical become one throughout the body. Because melanin behaves as a conductor in our bodies, antibiotics, processed foods, hormones injected in animals, alcohol, lack of sunlight, lack of foods found in nature, and smoking destroys (deactivates) the melanin that regulates the organs in our bodies. Each organ functions according to rhythm and that rhythm is controlled by the pineal gland. Again, a higher concentration of melanin causes people of color to require a higher amount of vitamins and minerals. That means more raw fruits and vegetables. A person of color that continuously depletes their melanin will open themselves up to disease two times more than a person of European descent. You are consuming the standard American diet and you are not American people. Not by blood.

You have African in your blood which means you have to maintain a natural foods diet for optimal health. "High blood pressure, stress, and hypertension are usually caused by a lack of proper nutrition. Improper nutrition weakens the internal organs, immune system, and lowers the organs' abilities to utilize nutrients, which feed the body."[38] Everything in the body that is not needed in a moment of crisis is shut down. In a stressful situation, your adrenal glands, located above your kidneys activate to defend you.

Your digestive system shuts down because it is no longer needed in true crises since you're not eating food. The digestive system is where you get the nutrients and energy from in the particular crisis and since no nutrients are being taken in, it relies on the nutrients already present in the body to get you out of the situation. Those nutrients can only be present if you are on a natural whole foods diet consisting of water, vegetables, fruits, quinoa etc. If your body is constantly being fed white sugar or white flour, it will create the same nutritional condition as stress because it robs your body of the nutrients (vitamin B, calcium, and vitamin D) you need to get though a stressful situation.

High salt (sodium) consumption overtime can become dangerous. Excess salt causes the body to retain water in the cells, which can lead to edema (swelling caused by excess fluid trapped in soft tissues). When there is excess salt in the body, the kidneys work with the liver to release an enzyme called angiotensin that increases your blood pressure. Once your blood pressure is increased, the adrenaline hormone is released (from the adrenal glands) to increase your heart rate. That's why you're at a higher risk for heart disease once you have high blood pressure. The body's demand for more nutrients in the blood causes the increase in pressure, which is the body's natural response to feed itself. "Wild animals produce more adrenaline and are under more stress and they do not have diseases associated with stress because their diet is raw food." Dr. Llaila Afrika

If high blood pressure is left untreated, the arteries can become hardened and less elastic, making it difficult to carry an adequate blood supply to the organs. This can lead to stroke, heart failure, kidney disease or hemorrhages. Everyday you're putting 87 (regular) in a body that requires 93 (premium) fuel. You can't do what less melanated people do because melanin reacts differently to certain chemicals in the body.

There is an interconnectedness throughout the body between the organs, blood, arteries, and nerves. Western doctors will typically turn to drugs as the solution to high blood pressure. This is a business and healing you takes money out of their pockets. The goal is to keep you comfortable with your dis-ease while you're making routine trips to the pharmacy weekly, monthly, or yearly. Certain blood pressure medication works by inhibiting the release of angiotensin. This is not solving the problem, it is masking the problem. If you want to reverse your dis-ease and come off of medication, then you must change what you're doing right now.

Along with diet, we have to minimize stress or change how we react to it. In holistic practice, if you carry fear, hurt, anger, envy, or hate in your heart, that too will obstruct blood circulation and create dis-ease in your body. Stress is known to be the source of all kinds of physiological dis-ease in the body, but as I have learned, if your body is equipped with the right nutrients, it can prevent issues for a while, but you still have to deal with the source if it is in fact stress; that will be covered in section three. The goal is to have spirit, mind, and body in balance to reverse any disease.

Something to assist with hypertension is to cleanse of course. I would suggest a raw food cleanse of twenty-thirty days that is mentioned in Chapter four. The Black and Latino community have a tendency to destroy food with salt. The issue with that is our taste buds have become so dull from all the over processed unnatural foods, that we have to over salt and over season everything. Now it is time to reset your taste buds. Eliminate caffeine, sodas, artificial juices, and caffeinated teas. Caffeine provokes the stress response which stimulates adrenaline production to shoot your heart rate up. Not only that, it is highly addictive and alters our heart, brain nerves, muscles, and mood.

From there, you would pay attention to how you combine your foods and increase your intake of raw fruits and vegetables. One thing I will mention is that cayenne pepper is known to dissolve blood clots and even stop heart attacks. That is because this pepper breaks down plaque, making your blood less thick. Adding a pinch to your food is highly recommended along with eating broccoli, parsley, kale, spinach and raw celery!

---

34. Pookrum, Jewel. *Vitamins & Minerals from a to z*. A&B Publishers Group, Brooklyn, New York (1999), Pg. 8

35. Afrika, Llaila O. *African holistic Health.* Buffalo, New York (2004), Pg. 58

36. Llaila O. Afrika. *The power and Science of Melanin; The biochemical that makes black people black.* Indianapolis, Indiana (2014), Pg. 12

37. Afrika, Llaila O. *African holistic Health.* Buffalo, New York (2004), Pg. 80.

38. Afrika, Llaila O. African holistic health. Revised 4th edition, A & B Books Publishers, New York (1993), Pg. 36.

10

SUGAR & SHIT

Diabetes is the number three killer of Americans. I don't want to go into separating all the diseases that are of the blood due to nutrition because the way to reverse them is quite similar. As you should have guessed by now, African Americans have the highest rate of diabetes compared to other ethnic/racial groups. The normal blood sugar range for white people is 80 to 120. Dr. Afrika tells us that black people get diabetes in the normal range (90) for white people because of melanin.

This harmful product called white sugar damages and weakens the immune system. Excess sugar overworks the pancreas, similar to how excess salt overworks the kidneys. Your pancreas is part of the digestion process. It creates juices to help break down foods while producing hormones to control the amount of sugar in the blood. White sugar is the worst possible sugar you can put in your body. It is literally over processed, stripped, and bleached shit made from sugar cane and bone char. Bone char is derived from cattle bones after burning them to ashes, which helps sugar achieve its white color through an absorption process. White sugar has no fiber, no nutrients, and increases the sugar level in the body leading to nutrient deprivation.

White sugar has the same addictive effects on the brain as cocaine or any kind of drug. High fructose corn syrup is extremely dangerous to consume because it goes into the bloodstream undigested which causes spikes in blood sugar and insulin. The liver alone can metabolize fructose, and as we learned earlier, anything deemed poisonous goes to the liver for filtration. Constant consumption of HFCS can lead to gout, high blood pressure, and insulin resistance in the liver.

"White sugar robs the body of minerals and vitamins, especially vitamin E. This robbery results in drowsiness, temper outbursts, hyperactivity, mood swings, tantrums, mischievousness, delinquency, laziness, and violence."[39] When you think about a fruit in its natural state, such as an apple, it contains natural sugars, vitamins, minerals and water. White sugar has no nutrients so when it is ingested, your body's natural tendency is to look for vitamins and minerals elsewhere. When it can't find any from this concentrated sugar it begins leaching the calcium in the bones to maintain the body's alkaline pH levels. Brown sugar is just white sugar coated in molasses, so you must avoid that too. Just think about what candy, sweets, and sugar do to our hard teeth. So what do you think it is doing to our soft tissues and organs over time?

Let's think of your liver and muscles as a night club. The insulin is the bouncer that lets too many people (sugar) in because they gave him a 20-spot. Now the club (liver and muscle) is to capacity and the bouncer (insulin) wants more money, so he continues to allow more people (excess sugar) into the club. There are still people outside that are waiting to come in. What are we going to do with them? We stick them in the basement (fat cells) knowing it is illegal to have it occupied. When the basement is to capacity, the people in line remain outside (in the blood.) Over time, too much sugar in the blood makes one pre-diabetic. **The overloading of the liver is causing it to turn sugar into fat.** More than often, I am hearing about children five and up who are pre-diabetic. We cannot allow our kids to consume so much sugar in their little bodies, setting them up for a life of injecting artificial insulin in their body's daily.

The hormone insulin is secreted by the highly melanated area called the Islets of Langerhans in the pancreas, which gets damaged from excess sugar consumption. It is necessary for the metabolism of blood sugar. People with type 2 diabetes are able to produce insulin but sometimes they eat so much that their pancreas is unable to keep up with the demand to make the insulin. In a lot of cases with type 2 diabetes, overweight people who lost weight were able to reverse their dis-ease.

In type 1 diabetes the cells in the pancreas are totally wiped out. Insulin is necessary to move glucose from the blood to the tissues, which makes type 1 diabetics dependent on insulin shots. Type 1 diabetics are typically lean because they can't make insulin, so they can't store fat. I believe with a 100% natural foods diet and right mind it can reverse type 1 diabetes and your pancreas can be regenerated. Melanin dominant individuals have the power to regenerate any organ they want in half the time compared to any other race with the right mind and environment. You have a gift from God called melanin and it's time to make it work for you.

Chromium is an excellent supplement for diabetes as it enhances the action of insulin. It helps insulin transport glucose into cells, where it can be used for energy. On average, 200mcg of chromium are recommended a day, but for Type 2 diabetes, 1000mcg is recommended split two to three times a day. Verify with a medical practitioner. Take the supplement with a plant-based protein, as it makes minerals (chromium) easier to transport from blood to cell.

If you are diagnosed as pre-diabetic and your physician is not working with you to set up a new diet and exercise plan, you need to RUN! The reversal to get your body back to balance is fairly simple and just requires discipline. Do not allow the doctors to put you on n cation for pre-diabetes. They are addicted to selling you drugs and are addicted to sugar. Bilberry herb and Chickweed are excellent h to help with cravings. We can't expect the doctors to solve all of our problems, so we need to completely obliterate our addiction with a new lifestyle. You can do it!

Remember carbohydrates like rice, flour, and pasta turn into sugar when processed by the body. We need to consume more vegetables, fruits, and unprocessed grains to reverse dis-ease. You will see the list of grains that aren't artificial on my food shopping list. There are those who are genetically predisposed to diabetes or high blood pressure. Fortunately, studies done in 2011 by The Norwegian University of Science and Technology showed over 75% of our diseases are controlled by what happens inside and outside of our body.[40]

There is a field called epigenetics that explains how changes in gene activity can occur without changing our actual DNA. Another study on 254 participants in Quebec also concluded that gene expression was different according to dietary patterns which can reduce the risk of chronic diseases.[41] Nutrition can influence our genes without changing their basic structure along with change in diet. Raw/pigmented foods help regenerate melanin through the nerve cells. This is especially important in men due to diabetes causing erectile dysfunction from poor circulation. In order for us to be in alignment with the rhythm of our body's chemical make-up, we have to start eating foods that will stop disrupting the harmony inside of us. Genetics do not predetermine health!

Whatever we put faith or belief in will become our reality. There are people I know that always say "its flu season", "its cold season", or "that runs in my family" so your automatically expecting the dis-ease to arise. We need to put forth belief that there is nothing wrong with the particular organ and must not call on dis-ease due to a weather, season, or time-frame. Cleanse yourself of poor food choices along with a negative mind frame that is always waiting to acquire dis-ease for whatever the reason may be. You are the strongest people on this planet and it's time for you to start believing that for yourself so you can take back your good health.

The body is a similar to a car. If you put premium gas in the vehicle, get your oil changes, breaks done, replace rotors, and basic maintenance- it will self-correct. Your body was designed to repair or destroy damaged cells, given the right environment. Fruits and vegetables contain phytonutrients, and these natural chemicals assist the melanin molecule with maintaining the health of our organs. Phytonutrients remove toxins out of the body by binding with them, protecting the cells from cancer causing agents, and can kill cancer cells.

I want to paraphrase a study that was done with twenty African Americans and twenty rural, black South Africans. Both groups switched diets for two weeks. The South Africans switched to a diet of burgers, fried chicken and potatoes while the African Americans switched to a traditional, local diet high in beans and vegetables. After the two weeks of a high fat, animal protein and low fiber diet, the South Africans had significant changes in their biomarkers (test to measure various areas of health) that indicated colon cancer risk while the traditional diet biomarker for colon cancer in the African Americans was greatly reduced.[42]

Remember keeping a balance between fruits and vegetables allows for optimal functioning of our organs. We are not in an environment that supports our genetic make-up, so we have a lot more work to do if we live in the Northern hemisphere. Raw foods are essential when reversing dis-ease because they are alive and will not require excess energy from our bodies to breakdown and digest. In order to ' ... , we must introduce foods into our body to induce healing. With her ... , supplements, and a whole foods diet, an overly acidic body can be ... out of an inflammatory and toxic state. Inflammation is the body's natural defense to fight infection. When the body doesn't turn off the inflammation response, healthy cells get attacked and can form disease. I myself do enjoy treats from time to time, but in extreme moderation due to the effects they have on the body.

OMIT IMMEDIATELY IF YOU HAVE OR ARE PRE-DISPOSED TO HIGH BLOOD PRESSURE OR DIABETES:

- SODA

- ALCOHOL (which is basically sugar)

- MEAT

- SALT (ESPECIALLY TABLE & MSG)

- PICKLES (all fermented foods)

- SMOKING

- VINEGAR (too acidic for an overly acidic body)

- COLD CUTS

- SOY (which is an anti-nutrient that depletes the body of iron and oxygen)

- DAIRY

- KETCHUP

- WHITE FLOUR PRODUCTS

- COFFEE (depletes body of serotonin which leads to depression and stress)

- HIGH FRUCTOSE CORN SYRUP (also named fructose as a cover-up)

HUMAN BODY REPAIR TIME:

- RED BLOOD CELLS – Approximately every four months

- BONES – Every ten years

- LIVER – Every 300 days

- SKIN – Approximately every three weeks

- LINING OF STOMACH and INTESTINES – Every five days

SMOOTH SKIN

Every KitKat, soda, artificial juice, doughnut, and bagel adds toxins to your blood that will greet you on your face or body as a pimple. Junk food and stress mess up hormone balance and increase inflammation. In holistic science, puffiness and dark circles under the eyes means there is dehydration and poor circulation, which can be related to weak kidneys. Water keeps skin hydrated and collagen plump. When the body becomes dehydrated the skin is the first organ to be starved of water.

Vitamin D encourages new skin cell growth and proliferation. Lucky for you, standing outside and absorbing the sun produces vitamin D2 in the liver of melanated people. Vitamin C is great for repairing connective tissue under the skin. You can get it from foods such as strawberries, kale, kiwi, bell peppers, and hibiscus flower.

When there is a break-out, it means your pores are clogged. Your skin is also an elimination organ, so acne is your skin taking a hot dump.

Moisturizer: I keep it simple because a lot of these overpriced cosmetics are contaminated with cancer causing agents and several known carcinogens. Once you cleanse your body, you won't be dependent on a variety of moisturizing agents. That's why you need all this junk, so your face doesn't feel like its cracking. Nevertheless, after I wash my face with black soap, I use a cotton ball and wipe my face with rose water or alcohol free witch hazel. My daily moisturizer is either African shea butter, jojoba oil, grapeseed oil, or vitamin E oil. I use Shea butter more in the winter months because it's thick.

To make your own moisturizer, you can add 70% shea butter, 20% carrier oil (jojoba oil) and 2% essential oil (lavender)

Mask: After a 10-minute facial steam (add three drops of lavender to steaming water), I make a mask of Bentonite clay or Moroccan red clay.

It pulls out toxins, draws out blackheads, chemicals, and heavy metals out of your pores. I even drink 1 teaspoon in ½ a glass of water for an internal flush, followed by a coffee enema. Combine 1 tbsp of bentonite clay, 1-2 tbsp of filtered water, 1 tbsp of organic oats, ½ a lime, and 2 drops of essential tea tree oil. Stay away from the eye areas. Mix together and try to get a nice consistency. You may have to add more water or clay but that's okay. Allow to dry for 20-30 minutes and take this time to lie on the floor with your legs up the wall in a 45 degree angle. Practice deep breathing and relaxation. Maybe put 2 cucumber slices over your eyes. Just take this time to relax. Do this once a week.

HERBS TO ASSIST WITH SKIN:

- **Bladderwrack:** is an antibacterial herb that inhibits breakdown in the skin while improving elasticity. It's rich in calcium, magnesium, and potassium. You can find it in capsule form, tincture, or drink as tea.

- **Skin Foods:** Apples, beets, blackberries, blueberries, dandelion greens, figs, grapefruit, kale, lemons, pears, watercress, cherries, coconuts, cabbage, and grapes.

- **Skin Tea:** Mix loose herbs of burdock, dandelion, nettle, red clover, lemon balm herb, and calendula. 1 tablespoon of each herb added to boiled water and steeped for 4-6hrs. Drink daily.

Other skin care techniques:

Skin brushing is using a brush with coarse bristle to brush dead skin cells off of the entire body. Skin brushing is also great for circulation! Don't forget saunas to drain out your lymphatic system, and seaweed/ ginger baths are great for the skin too. Steam your face once a week for ten minutes and add three drops of lavender to the water.

39. Afrika, Llaila O. African holistic health. Buffalo, New York (2004), Pg. 191.

40. https://nutritionj.biomedcentral.com/articles/10.1186/1475-2891-12-24 (2013)

41. Axe, Josh. *Eat Dirt; why leaky gut may be the root cause of your health problems and 5 surprising steps to cure it.* HarperCollins Publishers, New York (2017), Pg. 68

11

INFLAMMATION PROTECTION

WINNING LOTTERY NUMBERS

There's a special number associated with carbohydrates that advises us on what foods take longer to break down into glucose. Essentially how much each food increases your blood sugar. This number is especially important for diabetics. If you want to lose or maintain weight, it makes sense to get familiar with the Glycemic Index (G.I.). The glycemic index is a measure of how rapidly the carbohydrate in a food is absorbed into the bloodstream.

The three basic forms of carbohydrates are fiber, starches, and sugar. When you eat or drink something with carbs, your body breaks these down and turns them to sugar called glucose. Your pancreas helps regulate sugar in your bloodstream from the insulin it produces. We want to have more carbohydrates that will keep our body fueled and keep the blood glucose balanced.

Low G.I foods keep you fuller longer, while allowing you to eat less. High GI foods will shoot that glucose up to extreme levels and require the pancreas to produce a large amount of insulin. This makes you feel hungry even if you just ate. In the long run, this overworks the pancreas which can lead to Type II Diabetes. Check out the guide below to keep in mind what you need to consume on a regular basis versus what should be very limited or eliminated.

LOW GI: 1-55

Fruits: apple, pear, plum, prunes, cherries, peach, and oranges

Green vegetables: asparagus, arugula, avocado, broccoli, bruss sprouts, celery, broccoli, kale, spinach, cauliflower, eggplant, cha cucumber, mushroom, and zucchini

Beans: chick peas, lentils, lima beans, black eye peas, kidney beans, and peas

Grains: oatmeal, millet, bulgur, quinoa

MEDIUM GI: 56-69

Grains: brown rice, whole wheat

Fruits: pineapple, banana, prunes

HIGH GI: 70+

White bread, bagel, instant oatmeal, white rice, pasta, box, white potato, Glucose (dextrose, High fructose corn syrup, and grape sugar,) breakfast cereal, popcorn-**ANYTHING WHITE.**

Pre-diabetic persons can still enjoy fruits. Pay attention to the low glycemic index fruits.

WHAT THE HELL IS GLUTEN?

I never realized what a difference gluten made in foods until I bought gluten-free flour and had fried dumplings made with it. What a disaster! The dumpling would not hold its form and it was just terrible to eat as it was to look at. Gluten is a substance found in grains that give the dough its elastic texture. It is the glue that holds grains together. There are people who have gluten sensitivity and avoid it at all cost; but the way I understand how gluten works, it seems that it is an issue for almost everyone. We are all different, so some people can withstand the effects more than others.

Gluten contains lectins which are sticky molecules that are resis- to digestion and even to stomach acid. These molecules are so sticky they bind to our gut lining and interfere with our normal gut bacteria which leads to inflammation. When we are internally inflamed, more of the calories we consume are stored as fat and weight gain can occur. I have monitored people that I put on a "lectin free" diet when it seemed like a lot of other meal plans weren't working for them. They were able to lose weight along with healing themselves of ailments. Depending on your genetics your immune system can respond to lectins at a lesser or greater degree causing no issues or a host of issues.

Soybeans (soymilk/soy products) are high in lectins and interfere with absorption of essential minerals. "The trypsin inhibitors interfere with digestion that can lead to gastric distress, poor protein digestion, and an overworked pancreas."[42] Soy products also inhibit thyroid function which can lead to a host of dis-ease from maintaining weight to more serious dis-eases like cancer.

Gluten Free Grains: amaranth, flaxseed, brown rice, millet, buckwheat, oat, nut-flour, and quinoa

A Few Foods High in Lectins: Tomato, potatoes, dairy products, eggplants, winter squash, soybeans/soy products, sugar, cookies, pasta, rice, bread, flour, corn and peanuts.

Natural forming mucus in the body acts as a defense to trap lectins which causing inflammation. The more mucus you produce consuming these foods the more resistant you are to lectins.

*Okra is an excellent lectin remover if you still plan to consume these products.

Take home points:

- Corn has a high glycemic index and is high in lectins.

- Food sensitivities expand your waistline and lead to fluid retention, inflammation, and weight gain.

- Some people who cut out the foods that they are sensitive to lose five to six pounds within the first two week of removing foods from your diet.

_____

42. Gregg, Diana; The Hidden Dangers of Soy, Outskirts Press, Inc. (2008), pg. 37.

12

"LADY PARTS"

"You will see how the rest of your life
changes when your womb changes."

- QUEEN AFUA

WOMB-AN

The womb is a muscular organ in the pelvic region where the fertilized
egg develop. It is located approximately three fingers below the navel
and is attached to the fallopian tubes, which are pathways the unfer-
tilized egg takes to reach the uterus from the ovaries. When inside the
uterus, you see the myometrium which is the strong, smooth muscle
of the uterus. The cervix is the opening of the uterus and the vagina is
the muscular tube that goes from the cervix to the outside of the body.
The breasts are also part of the complex female reproductive system and
contain clusters of milk-producing glands called alveoli.

(See diagram below)

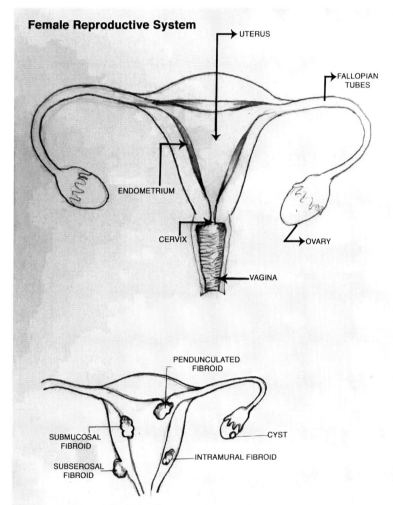

Female Reproductive System

UTERUS

FALLOPIAN TUBES

ENDOMETRIUM

CERVIX

OVARY

VAGINA

PENDUNCULATED FIBROID

SUBMUCOSAL FIBROID

CYST

INTRAMURAL FIBROID

SUBSEROSAL FIBROID

Different types of Fibroids (Treatment the same for all types)

THE RED SEA

Every month, a woman's body prepares for pregnancy. During a woman's menstrual cycle, her reproductive hormones make the eggs in the ovaries mature (ready to be fertilized by a sperm cell.) The hormones also thicken the lining of the woman's womb to provide a nice cushy landing for the egg if the woman does get pregnant. If pregnancy doesn't occur, the body doesn't need this thickened lining in the uterus so menstruation occurs; which causes the breakdown of the tissues and blood to flow out of the vagina.

"Menstruation is the loss of fresh blood, not diseased blood."[43] What I learned from my experience about menstruation in my early twenties is that excessive cramping and hemorrhaging are not normal. These conditions can be caused by unnatural foods, excessive animal meat, drugs, alcohol etc. I absolutely thought this was a normal part of womanhood until I performed a raw food diet. My periods used to last eight days with five days of extremely heavy bleeding. My cramping was so painful that I would roll around in my hallway until I got so drained and fell asleep. During menstruation women are losing calcium, thyroxine, magnesium, iodine, copper, zinc, vitamin B and E.

The diet I performed outlined in chapter three was for me to heal myself of chronic digestive issues, along with other issues the doctor wasn't able to diagnose. I did not do this cleanse because of my period. Reducing my period and eliminating cramps just happened to be one of the additional perks. It got to the point that I didn't even realize I was having my period. The length of my period was cut in half with two days moderately heavy followed by two lighter days. Woman who suffer with bleeding for more than five days do not need to suffer any longer. It is an unnatural lifestyle of processed, greasy, animal, salty and sugary foods that is suffocating your womb. "Over a period of twenty-one to eighty-four days, maintain a diet that consists of fifty percent green juices, purified or distilled water, and herbal teas specific to the symptoms of your womb experiences."[44]

To decrease the length of your period and the pain that accompanies it, you must decrease or eliminate your intake of animal protein, salt, sugar, white processed foods and dairy. The removal of these nutrient deficient foods should be replaced with green vegetables (raw or steamed lightly), leafy salads, beans and any foods provided on my food shopping list. Drinking a green juice with spirulina every day is very beneficial for womb rejuvenation.

Refrain from use of tampons because the waste is held in the vagina. Unscented sanitary napkins or the diva cup is safer. The diva cup is a cup that is to be inserted into the vagina and catches all the blood being released. After about six hours (every women's timing will be different) you remove the cup and pour the blood into the toilet. Aside from the fact that you get to see what's coming out of you, you'll also save a lot of money since the cup is reusable for at least one year.

FIBROIDS & CYSTS

"Fibroids can grow with or without a capsule. Inside the fibroid capsule, there can be rotten blood, trapped veins, arteries, cellular waste, and a mass of muscle or fluid pus. The tumor can be the size of a bean or as large as a grapefruit."[45] These little critters can be caused by a multitude of factors such as spermicide gel in condoms, acidic sperm, tampons, diabetes, hair relaxers, skin bleaching creams, cosmetics, excess salt, sugar, deodorant, high blood pressure, birth control pills, and poor diet to name a few. These can cause waste build-up, impair the immune system, and weaken the uterus. "Hormones in milk have caused cysts, tumors, cancer, and early menstruation in girls, gender confusion and feminization of males in studies."[46]

Fibroids and cysts (pockets of tissue that contain fluid, air, or other substances) are typically non-cancerous and do not require surgery. If there is an over consumption of unnatural foods along with these other factors, it makes it very difficult for the liver to neutralize the waste so it ends up building up in different areas throughout the body.

Traditional medicine often leans towards a hysterectomy as a solution to fibroids and cyst. Hysterectomy, which is the complete or partial removal of the uterus, is a common surgical treatment. There is a higher rate of hysterectomies performed on black and brown women as opposed to white women. The surgical procedure was performed throughout the nineteenth century by a monster named J. Marion Sims. This disgusting lunatic would perfect his "surgical techniques" on female slaves with no anesthesia because he felt women of color were more durable than white women.

The problem with hysterectomies is there's no guarantee the ailments won't return because the root causes were never addressed. This option has been offered to women close to me, especially the ones who have children already. They were told they don't need their uterus anymore and the surgery would alleviate these issues. The mere fact that a myomectomy (removal of the fibroid) wasn't offered as a solution to preserve the uterus should make you question these doctors. A hysterectomy is a short and easy surgery in comparison to a myomectomy which requires more skill. There are some doctors that would just prefer to give you what they know how to do rather than suggesting you find another doctor that can at least perform a myomectomy, allowing you the option to keep this vital organ of life.

I want you to understand that western medicine evolved from a male centered philosophy of European myths and superstitions. There were women in ancient Greece who were having issues with a prolapsed uterus. This means that after giving birth the uterus, rectum, vagina, and bladder became weakened and did not snap back into place. The wear and tear from child birth caused excessive sagging of the organs. The ancient method was to hang women by their feet from a ladder for a whole day and night assuming that gravity would pull their uterus back in place. Do you have a blank stare on your face yet? I'm not kidding. To add to this they place a peeled pomegranate into the vagina to hold everything in place! Granted we have come a long way from hanging upside down for a day but all physicians, their methods, and expertise must always be questioned.

All physicians "practicing" on patients for a particular issue eventually becomes the norm once the method is more common and easier such as a hysterectomy. It doesn't mean that it is the best way to solve the issue. The size of the fibroid does not matter, it can be removed through a bikini line incision, just like a ten pound baby can be removed from the same location. I'm only mentioning a myomectomy because there are some woman who will not want to go through the natural fibroid elimination treatment, but I don't want you to take your entire uterus out because it's better for your doctor!

There is no part of the body put there by accident, so in most cases, removing it won't correct all the issues and can set you up for hormonal imbalances later on in life. More importantly there are studies coming out that are linking a connection between the brain and the uterus. This means that a women's uterus may play a role in memory and cognitive functions. Professor Heather Bimonte-Nelson's studies showed that rats that had their uterus removed struggled more with their memory in a water maze than rats who kept their uterus.

As with most dis-ease in the body, stress-induced hormonal changes can lead to a wide range of issues. That stress coupled with a weak immune system is a recipe for disaster, so a full body cleanse is a must. It's not the stress that is the issue, but the reaction to the stress needs to be managed. In African spirituality, it is said that negative and toxic emotions associated with family, relationships, work, school or any life occurrences tend to be held in the womb if not dealt with appropriately. We must let go of all hurt lingering in our life so we can begin to heal our womb emotionally, physically, and spiritually. More on this is covered in section three.

FUN BAGS

"Overall, African Americans are more likely to develop cancer than persons of any other racial and ethnic group... African American women are more likely to die from breast cancer."[47] Can we be number one in something other than disease please? Breast cancer is a glandular cancer similar to prostate cancer, meaning the exit point of the glands are clogged with tumor cells. It is crucial that we eliminate the toxins, such as aluminum filled deodorants. The aluminum is not only toxic but designed to stop the body from its natural process of perspiration which keeps waste in the body.

The goal is to unclog the glands to allow for newly oxygenated blood enriched with vitamins, mineral and enzymes to reach the cancer cells and neutralize them. A cleanse is necessary for this to happen, whether it is a juice or raw food diet. While on this cleanse, a coffee enema should be performed three to four times a day as long as no chemotherapy has been done in the past.

Dr. Max Gerson was a German physician well known for healing cancer and other chronic diseases using Gerson therapy. This therapy focused on supporting the body's natural healing process through the use of natural elements. Gerson used fresh fruit and vegetable juices, flaxseed oil, B12 supplement, etc. to promote healing. "One of the most important techniques of the Gerson Therapy is detoxification via the liver/bile through the use of coffee enemas. Dr. Gerson knew that these dilate the bile ducts, thus allowing the liver to release toxic accumula-tions… rectal coffee administration stimulates an enzyme system (glu-tathione S-transferase) in the liver, which is able to remove toxic free radicals from the bloodstream."[48]

Once the cancer has been eliminated, maintenance of a natural foods lifestyle by at least 75% raw fruits and vegetables is key to helping the body stay free from dis-ease. The Gerson way of healing has proved to beat cancer a thousand times over. For more info on Gerson healing, check out the book, *Healing the Gerson Way,* by Charlotte Gerson with Beata Bishop.

Mammograms have also been linked with causing breast cancer. "The supposed increased risk of breast cancer from X-rays in annual mammograms has led to recommendations for women to avoid them altogether… Gofman estimated that 75% of breast cancers are caused by mammograms combined with other medical sources."[49] Routine mam-mography is recommended by the FDA, American Cancer Society, and National Cancer Institute. Cancer screening is a profitable business and it detects tumors only a year before they would have been found by self-touch breast examination. "When this year is subtracted from the sur-vival time of women who were treated after a mammographic finding, there was no difference in life expectancy compared with women who did not have mammograms."[50]

Bras are also linked with contributing to breast cancer. Ladies I know we want our breast up to our neck in that nice tight dress but we cannot wear them 24/7. "Lymphatic vessels are easily constricted by external pressure, such as from a bra. This compression prevents proper draining of the breast tissue, causing tenderness, pain, cyst, and finally, cancer. These breast problems are only found in bra-wearing cultures."[51] Conclusion to bras: Don't wear them while you're in the house or to bed. I have wireless or cotton sports bras that I wear throughout the day. Unless I am dressing up for an event, my boobs stay put!

HEART-BROKEN VAGINA

Most women will suffer from a yeast infection or bacterial vaginosis at some time in their life. "Bacterial vaginosis results from overgrowth of particular vaginal bacteria. The prevalence of bacterial vaginosis is higher in African American women."[52] Bacterial vaginosis (BV) can be caused by poor diet, prescription drugs, excess sugar, salt, and even a toxic man.

I had an experience where the normal balance of my lady part was disrupted every time I had a sexual encounter with the man I was seeing at the time, causing BV. He ate a diet high in processed foods, unnatural juices, Hennessey, soda, fast foods and also smoked excessive marijuana. Prior to gaining knowledge about natural healing, I would take the prescriptions from the gynecologist which never addressed the root cause; so the problem reoccurred. Ladies, I know sometimes we can feel ashamed of that not-so-nice scent or feeling that occurs with BV, but it's not always your fault.

Once this man changed his lifestyle to a natural diet, reduced his intake of meat, cut out fast foods, reduced smoking and started drinking water, the bacterial vaginosis stopped. What does this mean? A highly acidic penis can make your vagina very angry. You have two options, either have the penis change his diet or get rid of the penis. If the man is not the problem, then we have to look at ourselves. Poor diet, water, stress, smoking, and alcohol consumption, which is causing an overgrowth of bacteria, yeast and fungus that already live in the uterus. Women who eat poorly and lack exercise will continue to have these issues regularly. A vegetarian based probiotic is excellent to add to your daily regimen to help balance the vaginal flora.

Yeast infections can also be caused by poor diet and unbalanced vaginal flora. A normal vaginal pH is between 3.8 and 4.5, which is moderately acidic. This ph is maintained by having balanced levels of hormones and vaginal bacteria. This balance is crucial for maintaining optimal vaginal health. In my experience, birth control pills make yeast infections more likely by depleting important nutrients which weaken the immune system and throw the vaginal environment out of whack. When an imbalance occurs and the vagina becomes too alkaline, there's an overgrowth of bad bacteria which can cause a yeast infection.

THE "V" HEALING SHOP

Yeast infection diet: abandon sugar, white flour/food, and alcohol which yeast thrives on. Take a probiotic daily to balance out the "good and bad" bacteria. Refrain from sex, playing with yourself, lubes, or any unnatural products in your vagina. Generally, the vagina is more acidic which is hospitable to yeast and bacteria.

Yeast Herbs: ginger, garlic and pau d' arco. These can be used as teas

Topical: Shove a garlic clove right up there plain or wrap it in clean cheese cloth overnight. Give birth to the clove the next morning in the toilet.

Fibroids or cysts treatment: Do all treatments to aggressively eliminate fibroids/cyst.

- Clay (mud) packs - applied to the pelvic area. Mix 1 tbsp. of dry clay with enough hot, distilled water to make a paste. Spread the paste on clean cloth. I use cheese cloth. Place it on the pelvic area for up to three hours.

- Castor oil packs – pour castor oil onto gauze or cheese cloth and apply to the pelvic area with heat. You may leave it on overnight. I alternate between the clay and castor oil packs weekly.

- Liver flush – can also be performed when healing fibroids or cysts. Removing the accumulated toxins from the liver allows it to release more toxins stored throughout the body. See the liver flush recipe in remedy section.

- Natural foods diet - consumption of foods alien to our genetic make-up will create dis-ease. Eliminate all animal protein, as it has an affinity to bind to melanin molecules. Animal protein (especially chicken) has a tendency to make your ovaries stiff.

- Herbal combination 1 -(add 1 tsp. of each herb per cup of tea) - steep equal parts of red raspberry, black cohosh, blessed thistle, Chaste tree berry (vitex berry) and Damiana. Drink 2-3 cups daily to strengthen and tone uterus.

- Herbal combination 2 – combine equal parts of red clover, dandelion root, Echinacea, goldenseal, and burdock root. Drink 2-3 cups daily to cleanse blood and eliminate waste.

- **Glutathione** – 1000mg daily. Helps shrink the fibroid.

- Drink the juice of one lemon and two tablespoons of organic, black strap molasses daily. Molasses contains iron which is essential for its production of hemoglobin.

- "Fibroid green juice" – Mix equal parts of kale and dandelion, one cucumber, four celery stalks, two inches of burdock root, two inches of fresh turmeric, and one inch of ginger. May add half an apple if taste is too pungent at first.

- Take a hot bath 4X a week with 1 cup of Epsom salt and 10 drops of lavender oil. Soak for 20-30 minutes.

- Prayer and meditation – everyday take quiet time to focus/ visualize your uterus being healed

- Coffee enema – bring 32 ounces of filtered or distilled water to boil and add three tablespoons of organic, medium roast coffee. Boil for three minutes then reduce heat, then allow the coffee to simmer covered for fifteen minutes. While waiting for the coffee to cool, eat a piece of fruit to activate your digestive system. Once the coffee feels warm, strain it into the enema bucket (I use a cheese cloth lined in the strainer to prevent coffee grounds from getting in the bucket). Lay on your right side and insert two inches of the enema tube in your anus and breathe deeply. Once all the coffee flows into your rectum, hold it in for twelve to eighteen minutes.

"The body's entire blood supply passes through the liver every three minutes, carrying poisons picked up from the tissues."[53] I purchased my enema kit on Amazon.com and it came with a stainless steel bucket with all the necessary hoses.

Vaginal steaming is an ancient remedy that allows the steam from specific herbs to softly permeate the exterior of the vagina. **Vaginal steaming** is known to:

- Reduce discomfort with the menstrual cycle

- Decrease menstrual flow

- Detoxify emotionally

- Increase fertility

- Speed healing and tone the reproductive system after birth

- Assist with healing of menopause

- Not recommended if you have an IUD or during menstruation

Be sure to do vaginal steaming at least four times a month. You can make the herbs for the steam yourself, but my steaming specialist, Noni, also provides quality herbs, steaming gowns and stools at www.wombmenthings.com. Visit her site for herb combinations or to purchase directly.

I have rid myself of and assisted other women in reducing long, heavy menstruation, cramping, and eliminating ovarian cysts. My gynecologist wanted to surgically remove my cyst and I refused to go that route. I performed another raw food diet and continued juicing even after the month of raw foods was complete. I maintained a majority raw food diet that year. The following year when I went back for my check-up, the cyst was gone. I was also able to eliminate my fibroid.

Fibroids are prevalent amongst women of color for many reasons, one in particular being hair relaxers. I have been perm free for almost six years. When I first discovered the fibroids, I was pregnant with my daughter. I know going natural and learning to manage your hair can be very difficult, but it's worth it for the sake of our wombs. I have the coarsest hair you can imagine, but I learned to manage it and I now love what I used to be ashamed of. Plus, I save thousands of dollars now that I don't relax my hair or put $500 hair weaves in every other month!

Take home points:

- Drink vegetable green juices every day

- Limit or eliminate processed foods, vinegar (all types), animal protein, soy, sugar and salt

- Herbal douche monthly or as needed

- Limit wearing tight pants

- Use natural deodorant

- Examine your breast monthly

- Wear cotton panties

- Go natural when you're ready to release your hair from the straight jacket of perms

- Sleep without a panty and bra

- For heavy bleeding take 1-2 tbsp of black strap molasses daily (can add the juice of one lemon to molasses)

---

43. Afrika, Llaila O. *African holistic health*. Revised 4th edition, A&B Books Publishers (1993), Pg. 250.

44. Afua, Queen. *Sacred Woman*. The Random House Publishing Group (2000), pg. 91.

45. Afrika, Laila O. *African Holistic Health*. Buffalo, New York (2004), Pg. 416.

46. Afrika, Laila O. *African Holistic Health*. Buffalo, New York (2004), Pg. 209.

47. Afua, Queen. *Sacred Woman*. The Random House Publishing Group (2000), pg. 90.

48. Gerson, Charlotte with Bishop, Beata. *Healing The Gerson Way*. New Edition (2013), pg. 125.

49. Kaufman, Joel M. *Malignant Medical Myths*. Infinity Publishing (2006), pg. 196.

50. Kaufman, Joel M. *Malignant Medical Myths*. Infinity Publishing (2006), pg. 204.

51. Kaufman, Joel M. *Malignant Medical Myths*. Infinity Publishing (2006), pg. 235.

52. Afua, Queen. *Sacred Woman*. The Random House Publishing Group (2000), pg. 70.

53. Gerson, Charlotte with Bishop, Beata. *Healing The Gerson Way*. New Edition (2013), pg. 163.

13

IF LOOKS COULD KILL

According to the global cosmetic products market, the year 2017 was valued at 532 billion dollars. In just the 1st quarter, Ulta reported sales reaching $1.5 billion in the United States alone.[54] As astounding as these numbers sound, we are paying top dollar to apply toxic substances on our bodies. "The fact is that up to 60% of all substances sprayed or rubbed into the skin are promptly absorbed and travel straight into the bloodstream."[55]

Today's cosmetics are pumped with toxic chemicals such as SLS (sodium lauryl sulfate), which is a detergent that irritates the eyes, brain and heart. This chemical is used to degrease engines and clean floors. If you look at the ingredients in a majority of shampoos, hair relaxers, and face wash, you are sure to see this known carcinogen.

Every year I'm required to take a training course called OSHA. One of the many purposes of this course is to train employees about the dangers of working in or around certain hazardous substances. One of the many substances we are warned about is talc, which contains asbestos like material.

"As long as the man is not disabled, it is felt that he shouldn't be told of his condition so that he can live and work in peace, and the company can benefit by his many years of experience."[56] This was a remark made by Dr. Kenneth Smith in 1949 regarding mill workers whose chest x-rays showed early signs of asbestosis. To protect the interest of the company, this information was withheld from the employees.

Asbestos is a toxic ingredient commonly found in talc that causes cancer, respiratory issues, fibroids, cysts and tumors. This mineral talc is used in cosmetics and gives make-up its soft, silky feel. In 2018, the Johnson & Johnson Company was sued and paid nearly $4.7 billion to 22 women and their families that blamed the talcum powder in the products contributed to their ovarian cancer.[57] Johnson & Johnson is holding firm on their belief that talc does not contain asbestos. Could it be because they have the largest share in the talcum powder market? Maybe.

Other names we should be aware of when purchasing cosmetics or toiletries are:

Alpha hydroxyl acids, albumin, diethanolamine, tallow (animal fat), aluminum, kaolin, mineral oil, parabens, formaldehyde, para-phenylenediamine, sodium chloride, placental extract, sodium laureth ether sulfate, PEG (polyethylene glycol), and fluorocarbons. For a full list of toxic, cosmetic ingredients and their purpose, check out the revised and expanded book, *African Holistic Health*, by Dr. Llaila O. Afrika, pg. 228.

Once in a while, I do apply a little foundation or lashes if there is a special occasion. Due to the active ingredients in the products, I make my skin care routine very simple, which you can find in chapter ten. Remember, what you put on your skin, you're eating. Would you eat any of these products above?

54.https://www.forbes.com/sites/pamdanziger/2018/08/06/sephora-and-ulta-are-on-a-collision-course-then-there-is-amazon-where-is-us-beauty-retail-headed/amp/

55. Gerson, Charlotte with Bishop, Beata. *Healing The Gerson Way*. New Edition (2013), pg. 43.

56. https://www.asbestos.com/featured-stories/cover-up/

57. www.nytimes.com/2018/12/19/business/johnson-johnson-baby-powder-verdict.amp.html

14

"DEEZ NUTS"

"Food is not just vitamins and minerals, food it
is spiritual. Food seeks spirituality through us
and we seek spirituality through the food."

- DR. LLAILA AFRIKA

Most men know how to use their penis in the bathroom and in the bedroom. But some have no idea what's happening internally with their penis during both of these processes. So just like we did with the digestive system, let's view the diagram below of the male reproductive system below and learn the importance of the prostate gland.

"DEES NUTS"

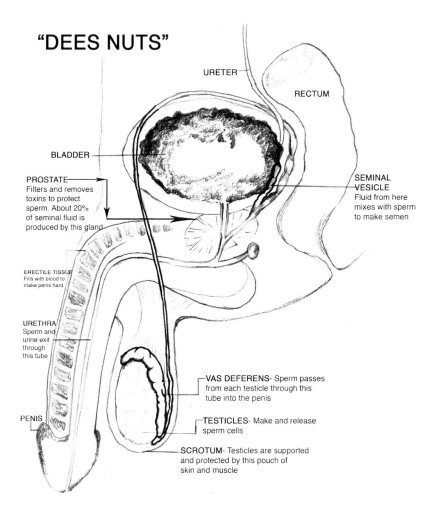

URETER

RECTUM

BLADDER

PROSTATE
Filters and removes
toxins to protect
sperm. About 20%
of seminal fluid is
produced by this gland

SEMINAL
VESICLE
Fluid from here
mixes with sperm
to make semen

ERECTILE TISSUE
Fills with blood to
make penis hard

URETHRA
Sperm and
urine exit
through
this tube

VAS DEFERENS- Sperm passes
from each testicle through this
tube into the penis

PENIS

TESTICLES- Make and release
sperm cells

SCROTUM- Testicles are supported
and protected by this pouch of
skin and muscle

The prostate gland is located directly below the bladder, and the rectum is behind the prostate, making it possible to feel the gland from the rectum with the finger. Don't get nervous now, I'm just giving you the location. During a physical exam, your doctor will check each testicle for lumps, tenderness, or change in size (you can also do this yourself). The doctor will also insert his/her finger into your rectum to feel the prostate for its size and any suspicious areas. This usually doesn't happen before age forty, so don't let this be the reason you don't go to the doctor.

A routine physical exam for men usually includes testing the blood pressure, taking the height, weight, testing for sexually transmitted diseases, and testicular cancer. Don't be one of those guys that only goes to the doctor when something is wrong. You should provide the same maintenance to your body that you would a Rolls Royce or McLaren.

The prostate is a muscle and a gland with several functions. Its primary function is to secrete and produce some of the alkaline seminal fluids during ejaculation. The prostate fluid, which is a whitish milky color, helps the sperm survive and protects them and the genetic code they carry in the acidic vaginal environment. The prostate fluid makes up about 30% of the fluid ejaculated and the rest is sperm and fluid from the seminal vesicles. The seminal vesicles are attached to the prostate and add extra fluid to the semen before it is sent down the urethra. The prostate erection nerves trigger the penis to swell and harden with extra blood flow into it, producing an erection. Sexual and reproduction tasks are highly dependent on the penis's blood vessels.

To function properly, the prostate needs the male hormones, testosterone and DHT- dihydrotestosterone. You know that face you guys make when you're about to ejaculate? The one that looks as if you're about to cry while being possessed? Here's what's happening…

The muscles of the prostate ensure that the semen is forcefully pressed into the urethra and then expelled outwards during ejaculation. The prostate contracts during ejaculation (sperm is travelling along two tubes called vas deferens), closing off the opening between the bladder and urethra and pushing semen through at speed. This prevents semen from entering the bladder and it's also why it's impossible to pee and ejaculate at the same time.

This important gland is responsible for filtering and removing toxins to protect the integrity of the sperm which promotes impregnation. There is a growing epidemic of prostate disease and cancer that is heavily due to a malfunction in this system. The enzyme

5-alpha-reductase converts the testosterone to DHT. Testosterone is the most abundant male hormone and DHT is the more active form cellularly. This conversion is extremely important because it is responsible for penile function and sex drive. Over time, toxins from the diet and environment can build up in the prostate gland, which may affect the production of 5-alpha –reductase and disrupt hormone balance.

MAN-BOOBS

Men with high estrogen levels and unbalanced male hormones are at risk for numerous ailments aside from prostate issues. These include arthritis, high blood pressure, baldness, low sperm count, diabetes and even dry skin. As discussed earlier, diet plays an important role in hormone production and balance. Conventional meat and dairy products are also heavily concentrated in dioxins (highly toxic compounds) which are known to cause cancer, infertility, and birth defects, etc. Mass-produced dairy has a "recombinant bovine growth hormone," injected into lactating cows to ensure constant milk production.

This hormone, along with hormones present in in-organic meats and factory foods, irritate your system and can cause man-boobs and malfunctioning of many organs, including the penis. Impotence and infertility can arise and the conventional method of treatment is to prescribe Viagra, Cialis, and Stendra. These pills have serious side effects, can lead to lifelong dependency, and do not address the core issues. In addition, as I mentioned in earlier chapters, prescription drugs do not get eliminated completely, and can remain in your body for ten to forty years...Maybe more.

It may be difficult for some to completely abstain from conventional meat and dairy but moderation is highly recommended. If you do have issues with getting an erection, don't forget to try either a fast, juice diet, or raw food diet which can help reverse the dis-eased state that the prostate gland is in. A weak body produces weak sperm. Seriously, do you really want to be that guy whipping out a penis pump or popping pills while your lady isn't looking?

Your body's design features an interconnectedness that you can't run away from. What you put in your mouth goes to your penis. Have you ever been with a woman whose vagina smells like sanitation? She takes a shower, but as soon as she is turned on, there goes that scent again. What she puts in her mouth, she puts in her vagina. It's the same thing for both sexes. Men have prostates – women have uteruses; Men have testicles – woman have ovaries; Man has penis – woman have clitoris. "The men's cycle closely duplicates the women's cycle. During a 28 day cycle, the man's sperm is triggered for ejaculatory preparation by hormones. The hormone balance changes in characteristics between the 14th and 28th day to stimulate sexual intercourse... At the end of the sperm cycle the sperm deteriorates."[58] What does this all mean? That men have a "period" too. We are alike and must care for our private parts the same way.

On the topic of sperm, I would like to share something with you regarding melanin when the sperm meets the egg. As Dr. Ann Brown notes in her lecture, Melanin is the foundation from which the cells of our bodies originated. Within the first three days after conception, something called a neural crest forms. This neural crest is responsible for producing our entire nervous system, spinal cord, nerves, brain, etc. A properly formed neural crest is dependent on the presence of melanin.[59] The eyes in a baby at just 35 days old are pure melanin. When you have an abnormal amount, you can get neurologic defects, retardation, cerebral palsy, etc. Your health and melanin content affects your ability to conceive a healthy baby – at the time of conception – which all ties back to your mental health and diet.

"We are living in a system that is not serving us to be our best."

−DR. JEWEL POOKRUM

My final note about semen is one I find quite interesting, but seems alien in this day and age. Brothers, you use your blood supply to make semen. Every time you have a jerk-session you lose 1 pint of blood; which most men don't replenish nutritionally. Excessive ejaculation reduces vital elements in the body. Semen is composed of zinc, selenium, lecithin, calcium, etc., which are all vital elements that can be found throughout the body. More importantly excessive ejaculation decreases cerebral spinal fluid (brain cells). This fluid is responsible for new sperm production. By retaining the fluid, you can boost your immune system, energize the body, stimulate the pineal gland, and reverse aging. Our ancestors knew of all the health benefits to a man if he held back his semen and practiced "injaculation." A man reabsorbs the elements of the seminal fluid through his lymphatic system.

Basically, during sex, you bring yourself just to the point of ejaculation, hold the semen in as long as you can, and that will regenerate the organs of the body. Once you finally release, it will be nothing but nutrient-less fluid because you will have retained all the vital elements with the hold back method (injaculation.) Men have been known not to release at all when close to ejaculation, withholding all the fluids. As difficult as this sounds, I would love for men to start trying this. For more details about this method, you can research Mantak Chia, who is a healing master that teaches and practices this method.

BALDIES & FITTEDS

Fellas, I understand that early balding is an uncomfortable issue. Those steroids, hormones, and excess estrogen from the dairy, chicken and red meat are throwing that circadian rhythm we discussed in the melanin section off beat. These excess hormones and steroids are causing your physical growth to surpass your mental growth. It's similar to when you see twelve year-old girls with "double D's." That's not normal; it's excess hormones in the foods aging them at alarming rates.

In 2017, I researched a way to stimulate hair growth when my mate at the time had a very large bald patch. There is a way that can help you to not have to hide under those fitted caps anymore. Unless it goes with your fit. Aside from changing your diet and having green juices daily, there are two at-home concoctions you can prepare to rub on your scalp. In a 6oz bottle, add hyaluronic acid to be the base of the serum, then add emu oil. Next add liquid saw palmetto to the hyaluronic/emu oil mixture. Shake the bottle, apply it to your scalp and around the hair-line for ten minutes. Then wash it off. You can do this twice a week.

For a daily topical scalp solution, you can make another serum by mixing peppermint oil and rosemary essential oil. We rubbed this oil on his scalp daily after massaging his scalp. We also purchased what is called a "derma stamp." The stamp has hundreds of tiny needles and a handle. Wherever there is no hair growth, stamp that area to pierce through the thin layer of skin on your scalp. If the hair follicle is completely dead, meaning no black dot in the scalp, then it may be impossible to revive the hair. We noticed with the derma stamp, it would bleed a little, so we wiped it off and then applied the rosemary and peppermint oil mixture.

From what I remember, I think it took about four to six months for the bald patch to be completely covered with hair. For someone with half their head bald, this operation can become tedious.

Also hanging upside down for a couple minutes can reverse blood circulation into the scalp. Two for one special, so be sure to try that. With your head hanging off the bed or for double the benefits, in a handstand. Only if you know what you're doing! He did the head off the bed for a few minutes along with the scalp mixture and voila! The complete article with measurements of ingredients can be found on www. hairguard.com.[60] I honestly just winged the measurements and we were fine. So before hiding under a durag and fitted for the rest of your life, check out the article and give it a try.

STICK AND MOVE

Wherever there is life there is activity. My brothers, once we implement the right diet, then we can work on building muscle while eliminating fat. YOU CANNOT TURN FAT INTO MUSCLE. Your burn fat and build muscle. A few major reasons for exercising are:

- **Increased Endurance**

- **Decrease/Relieve Stress**

- **Increased Self-Esteem**

- **Burn Fat**

- **Improve digestion**

- **Increased Flexibility**

Your bodies were created to move, so if you have a desk job, you need to get up periodically, stretch, walk around, foam roll in the middle of the office and drink water. Men do not believe they need to stretch for some strange reason. Stretching is not only for women. If you have or are about to start a workout routine, you need to have strength and flexibility to prevent injuries. Everybody and their mother is complaining about back pain. Nine times out of ten, when you have an area of pain the root cause is somewhere else. If you have low back pain, chances are you have tight hips, hamstrings, quadriceps, or all three and the shortness of those muscles is causing a pull on your lower back.

Tight hip flexors can lead to your booty becoming underactive; which leads to your body recruiting the muscles of your lower back to carry the load your butt should be carrying. The same can be said for knee pain.

"I can't squat, I have bad knees." No, you have bad knees because you don't squat. Most men completely abandon their lower half and continuously work chest, back, biceps and triceps. Yes, ladies love a nice sculpted chest, back, and arms, but if it is being balanced by two twigs below, you're in trouble. If you are that man who neglects your lower half, you either have lower back pain already or are on the way to it. You need to work your entire body in order to have balance throughout. This includes your ass. A strong ass will improve your squat, deadlift and overall movement patterns.

Your glute muscles are developed more than less melanated people because we have a high application of melanin in those muscles. That is why most black/brown people have a round ass and less melanated people have what we call a long back or "NOSSATAL." That means "no ass at all." They lack melanin in that muscle and have to rely on heavy lifting to attempt to grow or shape their glutes. Gentlemen, no one will judge you if you're in the gym doing hip thrust unless they have no idea what they are doing.

At twenty-five, I used to have terrible knee pain. I knew I had to do something about it because when I went hiking, I was able to get up the trail, but when it was time to come back down – OMG! My knees completely gave out on me and I was practically being carried by my bestie, Natalie. Poor girl is only 4'11" and I am 5'8"! When I got back home, I went to the doctor and luckily, he was honest with me and told me that my knees were fine and I was just weak. He told me I needed to build the muscles around the knee (quadriceps and hamstring) if

I wanted the pain to go away.

Of course, I didn't listen and decided to take a nice trip to France with my girl, Deidra. It happened again! We had to take a cab all over Paris because I couldn't walk. So, I joined a CrossFit gym, learned the key movements to build muscle, and studied/practiced functional movement for a couple years. No pain in my body and ten years later, I feel great. I want to help you to help yourself before you end up in a similar situation.

A few basic things you should be able to do are: touch your toes, bring the heels of your foot to your butt, butterfly groin stretch (without your knees eight feet in the air), and squat to the ground with your chest up and heels not coming off the floor. If these moves are nowhere near possible for you, then it's time to foam roll and stretch.

You foam roll first to break up what is called connective tissue that is over your muscle. A foam roller is a hard Styrofoam tool that allows you to give yourself a massage. You foam roll before stretching to get rid of the knots in the body. We wouldn't want to stretch something that has a knot in it so deep tissue massage is very important and it balances the physical alignment. You should also have yoga or stretch sessions two times a week. If you don't stretch it daily, the connective tissue will begin to harden making it harder to break up later down the line. This is so important because we need the oxygen to be able to flow through our muscles while working out, stretching, and doing basic daily activities.

Hold the stretches anywhere from thirty seconds to one minute if you are a beginner. Before the workout, don't hold long stretches; just do a dynamic warm-up that mimics what you plan on doing for the day. Warm-up should be about ten to fifteen minutes. Stretch during the cool-down at the end when your muscles are nice and hot. I find PNF (proprioceptive neuromuscular facilitation) stretching to be the most affective. PNF stretching tricks your nervous system into relaxing so you can get more range of motion or length in your tissue. For more info on PNF stretching, you can check out a book called *Relax Into Stretch* by Pavel Tsatsouline. You can also find great mobility routines to do before your workout and stretch routines after your workout on YouTube. I also post routines on my Instagram so follow me for all that good stuff.

People all around the world want a flat stomach or abs and are doing all the wrong things to get it. Five hundred crunches a day will not give you great abs! Especially if there's a thick layer of fat hiding these muscles. The first thing is to get your diet in order so you can lower your body fat percentage along with exercise. You have a lot of options to change your diet to reduce your body fat in this book, so choose one and get started.

All these new machines and crazy looking exercises are unnecessary. Stick to the basics and you will get results. You always want to include moves that are unilateral (one side at a time) so you can pinpoint your weaknesses. You don't have to hang upside down on a pull-up bar by your big toe while doing side crunches. Here are a list of must-do, basic exercises to work on mastering weekly before hanging from a bar by your big toe. You can find a demonstration of these moves on YouTube but I highly suggest investing in a trainer. Never start a new program with weights. Master the movement first. If you have no interest in lifting weights then Yoga is a must! Strength, flexibility, and meditation all in one.

A FEW OF NEEK'S HOLY GRAIL OF EXERCISES

QUADS	HAMSTRING	CHEST	BACK	CORE/ABS	GLUTE	BI/TRI/CALVES
BACK SQUAT	CONVENTIONAL DEADLIFT	PUSH-UPS	PULL-UPS	PLANK	HIP THRUSTERS	DIPS
FRONT SQUAT	ROMANIAN DEADLIFT	BENCH PRESS	BACK EXTENSIONS	SIDE PLANK	PISTOL SQUAT	TRICEP EXTENSIONS
ALTERNATING FRONT LUNGES	SINGLE-LEG DEADLIFT	DUMBBELL PRESS	BARBELL ROWS	HANGING LEG RAISES	GLUTE BRIDGE	BICEP CURLS HAMMER CURLS
WALL SITS	REVERSE LUNGES	CHIN-UPS	DUMBBELL ROWS	RUSSIAN TWIST	FIRE HYDRANTS	CALF RAISE
BULGARIAN SPLIT SQUAT	GOOD MORNINGS	DUMBBELL FLYES	LAT PULL-DOWN	CRUNCHES	BULGARIAN SPLIT SQUAT	DONKEY CALF RAISES
WALKING LUNGES		DUMBBELL PULL-OVERS			BOX STEP-UP	
GOBLET SQUAT					SUMO DEADLIFT	

PROTEIN- PROTEIN- PROTEIN

Now my kings, I understand you want protein to build muscle, so you have a tendency to overindulge in animal protein. Animal protein may give your body strength, but it also accelerates the aging process and cell degeneration. Just because you can squat 315 pounds for twenty reps doesn't mean you're healthy.

Our ancestors ate a high protein diet, but it was plant-based protein. A high protein diet can be very acidic. Healthy blood and tissue pH should be about 7.3-7.4; urine and saliva pH 6.8-7.2. High protein diets can easily move you out of this range and cause burden on your kidneys as well as the rest of your internal system. In order to digest this high protein diet, your body begins to leach out minerals in the body and pull calcium and magnesium out of the bones, which can lead to brittle bones, joints, or osteoporosis down the line. Animal protein intake should be very moderate or none at all.

Excess animal protein accelerates the growth of cancer cells in the body. If still transitioning, please have grass-fed meat, free range chicken or turkey, and wild caught fish no more than three times a week. You don't really love meat, you love seasoning and fire. Animals that eat meat capture their prey and kill it, and then digest everything raw. They don't turn on their stoves, soak the meat in vinegar/lemon, season it with Lawry's (terrible), put it on the fire and stew it. They do not need to chemically alter what they are about to eat to ingest it. You have to because your bodies were not made to consume the amounts and types of meat we have on a regular basis. The chemicals found in non-organic meat and processed foods overwork your kidneys and liver. Eating meat makes you as plump as sugar does. Red meat and dairy products contains a sugar molecule called Neu5Gc (N-Glycolyneuraminic acid) which is linked to heart dis-ease and cancer. Reason being is the body suffers an immune reaction to sugar, which is a foreign substance in the body.

Protein from eggs is also an issue in excess, because the yolk is highly concentrated in saturated fat. Not good for someone with high cholesterol. Limit to two times a week if you're still transitioning out of eggs. Excess protein has a tendency to thicken the blood allowing for poor blood circulation; that's why you will still see very fit people with heart disease. Whey and casein protein also negatively impact our health because they come from dairy. There is no nutritional value left from cows milk once its pasteurized (heated up).

Great endurance doesn't equal great circulation. Remember, cancer thrives on every form of animal protein there is because it behaves as toxins in the body! The dirtier the meat, the better.

**Without doing everything perfectly, you
can still achieve progressive results!**

A few plant-based protein options that are easier to digest than animal protein:

- Quinoa/Amaranth – contains all 9 essential amino acids; ½ a cup has 14g of protein

- Lentils – 1 cooked cup has 18g of protein

- Raw spinach – 2 cups have 2.1 grams of protein

- Chickpeas – just half a cup has anywhere from 15-20g of protein

- Almonds – ¼ cup has 8g of protein

- Spirulina – (MY FAVORITE) contains 22 amino acids; just 2 Tablespoon has 8g of protein. Also known to build immune system and reduce blood pressure

- Chia Seeds – 2 Tablespoons have 4g of protein

- Hemp Seeds – ¼ cup has 15g of protein

- Broccoli – 1 regular size stalk has 4.3g of protein

- Ezekiel Bread – 2 slices of this sprouted grain has approximately 8g of protein

- Oats/Oatmeal – ½ a cup has approximately 6g of protein and 4g of fiber

Avoid: White sugar, alcohol, junk food, non-organic meat, eggs, dairy and salt

---

58. Afrika, Llaila O. African holistic health. Revised 4th edition, A & B Books Publishers, New York (1993), Pg. 233-234.

59. Brown, Ann. Published on December 17, 2012. "Melanin & Pineal Gland pt. 1." https://youtu.be/qYTfR60XsFU

60. http://www.hairguard.com/how-to-stimulate-new-hair-growth/

15

"LET FOOD BE THY MEDICINE"

Medical science has made some amazing discoveries, but there is no comparison to what's provided by nature. Nature is so intelligent that it put the medicine in the food. My sister, Samantha, was almost confined to medication from nine years old until it was time for her to leave earth. She came to the States from Jamaica at seven years old. At nine years old, she began to have chronic seizures, and naturally, my mother took her to the doctor to seek help. They went to a series of different doctors and it was the neurologist that told her she had a hole in her brain. But then the cardiologist told her she had a hole in her heart.

My sister's seizures lasted for around seven to ten seconds. But as she said, "It is the most intense seven seconds of your life; you have no control over your body. The drooling starts, your tongue shifts and you black out."

The scariest part was that she could feel when the seizure was coming so she would prepare herself for it. My brother and I witnessed her having a seizure in the dining room, and as scary as it was to watch, I can't even begin to imagine how scary it was going through it.

Unsurprisingly, the doctor recommended her to start taking all sorts of medication to, what I like to refer to as, mask the dis-ease. My mother did not want her nine year old to live with dis-ease or be made comfortable in it. She took my sister back to Jamaica to visit a natural healer named Bongohue, who would ultimately become my sister's savior.

My mother and my sister went to see Bongohue in a mountainous region in the country. He asked my sister what her favorite foods were, primarily what her diet consisted of. She remembered telling him that she loved pizza. Bongohue told Samantha she had to cut back on all the white stuff and dairy and provided her with "brown stuff in a Wray and Nephew bottle." My sister, even at nine years old, began taking her herbs in doses daily along with a change in diet.

From nine to ten years old, the seizures became more and more spaced out. By eleven years old, they were completely gone, and she never had another seizure again. Wow… let's give Nature a round of applause! Allopathic medicine treats nature as an assailant that must be restrained. Bongohue is a God to our family and my sister! He is a true healer… he is IMHOTEP.

THE REAL FATHER OF MEDICINE

IMHOTEP - meaning "The one who comes in peace," was an ancient Kemetic (Egyptian) Sage, High Priest, Architect, and a revered Healer. Aside from being Kemet's first known architect, he was the first to extract medicines from plants to heal. He did not add chemical compounds that are unnatural to the body as modern science does today. Imhotep is the original author of the Edwin Smith Papyrus and Ebers Medical Papyrus. Papyrus is an old material that our ancient ancestors recorded information on. On this Papyrus was information on anatomy, surgery, diagnosis, and treatment on an assortment of medical issues.

Interestingly enough, when you graduate medical school, you are supposed to take the "Hippocratic Oath." This oath requires new medical physicians to swear to multiple ethical standards. Hippocrates is referred to in the Western world as the "Father of medicine," but he lived from 460-377BC. The books by Imhotep are the oldest medical books in history and were written thousands of years prior to Hippocrates' birth.

Hippocrates' work is inextricably linked with that of our ancestor in Ancient Kemet. We were and still are the original healers, but as you all know, you won't get this information from our schools. You are all natural-born intelligent healers with the ability to help yourselves as well as your families. You all are just as great as Imhotep; you just have to tap into your super powers. As your body gets cleaner and the blood becomes purer, your awareness levels increase and mind opens up. As the old saying goes, "We are divine spiritual beings having a divine physical experience."

Now maybe you've read everything up to this point and still don't feel like you want to change. Well, then screw you! Just kidding J…I usually hear, "What's the point? I'm going to die anyway." The reason you feel this way is because you haven't discovered a deeper essence of your existence. We will find your purpose together by introducing you to a deep committed relationship with yourself so you won't feel that way. That will be covered more in the final section of this book.

I want to leave you with my personal food shopping list of items I like to have at home. I go to the market anywhere from one to three times a week because food from nature doesn't last that long. On this list, you won't find the first-class flight to your death-bed items. Those items are:

- Dairy (doesn't matter if it is organic)

- Fried Foods

- White sugar, Sweet "n" low, Equal, Truvia (not stevia), brown sugar and Splenda

- White flour products

- Cold cuts (stop giving your children these sandwiches!)

- Alcohol

- Energy Drinks

- Canned vegetables

- Foods containing corn or rice syrup

- Artificial sweeteners, flavorings or colors

NEEKS NUTRITION KITCHEN LIST

VEGETABLES	FRUITS	PROTEINS	GRAINS	HERBS/SPICES	MISC
Watercress	Blueberries	Free Range Organic Chicken	Quinoa	Turmeric	Hemp Milk
Arugula	Strawberries	Wild Caught Salmon	Amaranth	Pink Himalayan Sea Salt	Oat Milk
Spinach	Blackberries	Grass-Fed Beef (limited)	Bulgar Wheat	Cayenne	Pea Milk
Brussel sprouts	Avocado	Organic Free-Range Eggs	Brown rice	Cinnamon	Almond Milk
Kale	Raspberries		Spelt	Nutmeg	Date syrup
Bell Peppers	Dates		Ezekiel Bread	Oregano	Agave syrup
Dandelion Greens	Apples		Buckwheat	Thyme	Raw Walnuts
Bok Choy	Bananas		Whole Oats	Cumin	Raw Almonds
Radicchio	Grapes	*Vegan Protein*	Black Rice	Basil	Almond Butter
Cauliflower	Watermelon	Lentils	Millet	Rosemary	Coconut Water
Purple Cabbage	Papaya	Hemp Seeds	Wheat flour (limited)	Pure Sea Salt	Pumpkin Seeds
Green Cabbage	Cantaloupe	Chick Peas	Brown Rice Pasta	Ginger	Chlorella
Yams	Oranges	Spirulina	Farro	Curry	Coconut oil
Zucchini	Grapefruits	Almonds	Wild rice	Cayenne	Flaxseed
Eggplant (limited)	Lemons	Quinoa		Garlic	Tahini
Leeks	Limes	Chia		Sage	Grapeseed oil
Scallion	Peaches	Oats		Onion Powder	Olive Oil
String beans	Pears			Garlic Powder	Brazil Nuts
Onions	Pineapples	Fruits & Veggie cont....		Dill	Hempseed oil
Squash	Cucumber	Parsley		Old Bay	Seaweed
Celery	Tangerines	Green Banana		Bay leaf	Coconut sugar
Okra	Figs	Callaloo		Fennel	Stevia
Butternut Squash	Plums	Soursop		Tarragon	
Yams	Acai	Cherries			
Olives	Mangoes	Kiwi			

Shirley's must have natural herbs/ remedies for overall well-being

(I just wanted to give several options. This doesn't mean buy everything on the page)

Some herbs may repeated throughout the list do to their multiple functions.

*If the herb is the root or bark, it is to be simmered on the stovetop for 25-30 minutes, then strained.

*If the herb is a stem, leaf, or flower it is to be steeped for 20-30 minutes or more.

*Average combination of herbs is typically three, but no more than five herbs in one tea.

*Herbs can be taken in capsule or tincture form as opposed to tea.

Pineal Gland

- It is very important to activate the pineal gland to **stimulate melanin production** during all healing processes from dis-ease.

- Tea – (add 1 tsp. of each herb per cup of tea) – combine equal parts of Gotu Kola, Ginkgo, blessed thistle, Echinacea, and false unicorn.

- Foods that increase melanin production – Bananas, avocados, pumpkin seeds, flaxseeds, chia seeds, lima beans, lentils, black beans, chick peas, grapes, mushrooms, quinoa and kamut.

- Copper – assist with melanin production **but only needed in tiny amounts**. Can be found in sesame seeds, swiss chard, spirulina, cashews and almonds.

Circulation

- Cayenne Pepper – lightly sprinkle on food

- Ginkgo Biloba – also known to boost memory

- Vitamin E

- Ginger Root – helps get rid of mucus and circulates the blood

- Nettle – I drink the tea. It's also great for asthma, and allergies

- Coenzyme Q10 – is an antioxidant naturally present in the body (heart, liver, kidneys and pancreas) but production decreases as we get older. Assist with high blood pressure.

- Folic Acid – creates more red blood cells (rapid cell division and growth)

- Parsley Juice – rich in chlorophyll and absorbs oxygen in the blood stream

Stress

- Ashwagandha – This root strengthens adrenal, thyroid, and immune function. Decreases inflammation. Relives anxiety and PTSD. Also promotes sleep!

- Schizandra Chinensis – similar to Ashwagandha, used for sleep, energy, and vitality.

- Holy Basil – Calms, energizes, and balances blood sugar levels.

- St. John's Wort – treats mild to moderate depression.

- Lemon Balm – (I love this one) tea or capsules promotes brain function. Assist with anxiety, hyperactivity, insomnia, and wishy washy-moody people.

Digestive Tract Repair/inflammation relief

- Cascara Sagrada – laxative for constipation/ breaks up intestinal waste (give 6-8hrs for bowel movement). Add 4oz of Cascara Sagrada to 2qts of distilled water and let it soak for 8hrs. Then boil for 1hr. Strain and add more water to herbs. Boil again for 1hr. Combine both herbal tonics and have 1tsp. 3-4X a day.

- Ginger Root – reduces inflammation in the intestinal tract and has protein digesting enzymes.

- Fennel Seed – reduces gas, indigestion and can break up kidney stones and uric acid.

- Psyllium Husk – stimulates the intestines to contract and speeds passage of stool. Also eases constipation when combined with water; like chia seeds, it swells up and becomes slippery. **Must drink with plenty water.** If you take a teaspoon in 8oz of water before a meal, it will give you a full feeling while washing out the colon and small intestine.

- Slippery Elm Bark – Soothes colon and assists with inflammation.

- Olive Oil – take a teaspoon a day after you have your warm water and lemon (or before a meal.)

- Goldenseal – can drink tea or take in pill form.

- Moringa – An herb that comes in powder form in U.S., but the seed can be eaten alone if you can find it. It is well known in Jamaica for its nutritious content and anti-inflammatory/antioxidant properties.

- Rhubarb Root – softens stool to make taking a dump nice and easy.

- Peppermint Tea

- Digestive Enzymes – 20-30 minutes before you eat.

- Pineapple – contains bromelain, an enzyme that helps decrease inflammation. Taken on empty stomach assist with break down proteins.

Constipation
(chew your food thoroughly and eat more Fiber)

- Yellow Dock – great for tightening and toning the colon

- Turmeric – also supports healthy brain function.

- Lemon or Grapefruit

- Senna Leaf – (stool softener) Increases water and electrolytes in the intestines. Also activates muscle contraction of the intestines (peristalsis). This is not to be used on a regular basis as it can reduce the intestines ability to contract over time, making you dependent.

- Cayenne Pepper – sprinkle on foods.

- Colon Detoxifier – Psyllium Seed, Flaxseed, Chia Seed or Hemp Seed.

- Coffee Enemas – (Enema kit can be purchased on Amazon. com)

Stops overgrowth of yeast and bacteria. Removes parasites from the digestive tract along with heavy metals. (See Chapter 12 for instructions)

Heavy Metal Remover

- Activated Charcoal – Acts as a magnet for toxins, food additives, poisons, drug residue and removes it through the colon. I drink a teaspoon in 6oz of water at night to assist cleansing during sleep.

- Rhubarb Root – Binds toxins (heavy metals) in the blood stream.

Note: Aluminum and Fluoride are toxic heavy metals that can be found in toothpaste, pots, baking powder, foil, drugs, and pans. Aluminum toxicity can lead to, memory loss, weak muscles, bone loss, depressed liver and kidney function, and osteoporosis.

Common cold and weak immune system

- Elderberry – Treats cold, flu, and softens and removes mucus from the respiratory system.

- Echinacea – nourishes the immune and lymphatic system. Stimulates white blood cells/antiviral.

- Astragalus Root – this herb is rich in antioxidants, boosts immune system, and reduces stress.

- Vitamin C – double up when sick as your body tends to absorb it faster.

- Goldenseal

- Sarsaparilla – is anti-inflammatory that is effective for tumor reduction, muscle pain, indigestion, liver damage, fevers, bloating, sexual impotence, and psoriasis. Also binds with toxins for removal from the blood stream.

- Sea Moss – (Irish Moss) is known for its powerful anti-inflammatory effects. Great for digestive health, mental health, fertility, and thyroid support. Rids the body of mucus and is a natural decongestant.

Diarrhea

- No eating, just vegetable juices or chamomile tea

Sleep

- Ashwagandha, Valerian root, Blue Skull Cap, or Blue Vervain (Wild hyssop). (Choose one herb, can be taken in pill form or tea)

Acid Reflux

The return of acid into the esophagus from the stomach damaging the lining of the esophagus. Herbs that can help with this are:

- Milk Thistle

- Dandelion Root – assists in detoxification of colon, liver, and kidneys.

- Digestive Enzymes – 20-30 minutes before you eat.

- Fennel Seeds – Rich in essential vitamins and minerals, which are released and absorbed into the bloodstream when chewed. Chew seeds raw before and after meals, ½ a teaspoon. Also makes your breath nice and fresh J

Headache

- Inhale lavender or eucalyptus essential oil. Lie down with cool damp cloth over forehead and eyes.

- Green tea

Symptoms of Parasites

Aches and pains throughout the body, digestive issues, heavily coated tongue, hot breath, ulcers, and menstrual irregularities.

Heart Health

- Hawthorne Berry – Boil 1.5pints of distilled water, add 2oz of cut Hawthorn berries, 2oz of cut Motherwort herb to water; cover and steep for 15 minutes. Drink 2X a day.

Kidney Flush

- Organic REAL cranberry juice – not that Ocean Spray crap (water it down heavily.)

- Nettle leaf tea – Assists with kidney stones and urinary tract infections.

- Parsley Root

- Hydrangea Root – assist with dissolving calcium deposits in soft tissue. Also dissolves kidney stones.

- Golden Rod – is an astringent and diuretic excellent for dissolving stones in kidney/bladder. Put 1oz of golden rod leaves (cut) in distilled water and allow to sit for 2hrs Bring to boil, simmer for 20 minutes, strain and cool. Drink every 4 hours.

- Celery – Drains excess water from the kidneys.

A great juice to make at home is: 1 Cucumber, 4pcs of parsley, ½ cup of broccoli, and ½ a lemon.

Liver Repair

- Milk Thistle – eases inflammation and assists with cell repair up to 30% (great for heavy drinkers). It protects the liver from being damaged by toxins.

- Chickweed – is an herb that also helps with inflammation, asthma, constipation, and psoriasis.

- Ginger Root

- Turmeric

- Dandelion Root – assists in detoxification of the colon, liver, and kidneys.

- Yellow Dock Root

Gall Stones

Apples (pure apple juice is great), Dandelion greens, Grape Fruits, Parsley, Celery, and Goose berries.

Example Liver and Kidney flush tea: 2 tablespoons of burdock root, 2 tbsp. of yellow dock root, ½ tbsp. of sarsaparilla, 1 tbsp. of elderberry, ½ tbsp. of red clover. Boil approximately 2 cups of water. Pour over herbs and steep for 3 hours.

Example Liver Flush drink: ½ cup of lemon juice, 1 garlic clove, pinch of cayenne pepper, and ¼ cup of lecithin granules.

Kidney Flush Juice: ½ cup of lemon juice, ½ cup fresh squeezed grapefruit juice (not box juice), 1 garlic clove (juiced or finely diced), 1oz of ginger (juice fresh ginger), and a pinch of cayenne.

Blood Cleansers

- Burdock Root Tea – Detoxes lymphatic system and liver.

- Red Clover – aids lymph (fluid) flow and is a known blood purifier.

- Yellow Dock Root Tea – (Brace yourself for this taste)

- Sassafras – plant is effective against excess mucus discharge.

- Chaparral – anti-inflammatory, kills parasites

- Echinacea/Goldenseal

- Soursop leaf – This plant is found in Jamaica and is known for attacking and destroying cancer cells, healing gout, stabilize blood sugar in diabetes, boosts immune system and prevents infection. When I go to Jamaica, I make sure to bring the dried leaves back to make tea.

Ex Blood cleanse Tea: Bring 2 cups of water to boil then reduce fire. For 30 minutes simmer equal parts of: Burdock Root, Sarsaparilla, and Sassafras (2 teaspoons each.) Strain and drink.

Cancer treatment

- 100% raw food diet

- Boil 10 soursop leaves – in 3 cups of water until about 2 cups dry out. Strain and allow to cool. Drink every morning for 4 weeks. Soursop has the ability to move mucus and toxins out of the blood.

- Coffee enemas (see preparation in chapter 12)

- Turmeric – (curcumin) has scientifically proven benefits against heart disease, Alzheimer's and cancer because of its anti-inflammatory and antioxidant properties. It also contributes to healthy digestion. You can sprinkle the powdered version on your foods.

Prostate Issues

- Saw Palmetto – is an extract of the berry of the Saw Palmetto tree. Helps the body hold on to its testosterone while allowing the prostate to maintain its size. Meaning it assists with an enlarged prostate by reducing the activity of inflammation. Also known for its hair growth benefits in men.

- Maca Root – supports energy and vitality. Reduces symptoms of depression and anxiety.

- Echinacea

- Witch Hazel Bark – (Not the liquid used to clean the skin) Known to ease inflammation due to its anti-inflammatory properties. Also great for warding off viral infections.

- Muira Puama – the root and bark of this plant assist with sexual performance, improved erectile function.

- Pumpkin seeds, raw almonds, and sesame seeds

Balding

- MSM tablets, Nettle leaf tea, and Progesterone

- Sea Moss – (Irish Moss) is known for its powerful anti-inflammatory effects. It is loaded with potassium, iodine, iron, beta carotene (for eyes), protein, and calcium. Great for digestive health, mental health, fertility, and thyroid support.

The thyroid is especially important due to its role in immune function. The thyroid regulates the body temperature, namely the fever. A lot of people get very nervous when their body temperature goes over 98.7. A fever is your body's way of healing itself and you should know that most viruses, germs and malignant tissue do not survive in elevated temperatures. A well-functioning thyroid supplied with iodine helps restore health. Chlorine in the water supply is able to remove iodine from the thyroid. Fluoride, a dangerous toxin, is even more powerful in blocking this important element. Sea moss is a great natural way to supplement the body with iodine.

Sea Moss is one of the most nutritious foods on the planet. Rids the body of mucus and is a natural decongestant. My Jamaican people love Irish Moss, but I will show you a healthier way to prepare it so you get all the vitamins and minerals. The one you get at the "Yardie" Restaurant can be a treat once in a while, "but di ting too sweet fi drink all di time." (It is too sweet to drink on a regular basis.) SEA MOSS HAS 90% OF MINERALS YOU NEED IN THE HUMAN BODY.

Big Shirley's Irish Moss Recipe:

For preparation, you soak sea moss for several hours or a day with lime to clean off the "sea" residue. Remove it from the water and rinse well! Blend 6oz of Irish moss with 32oz of purified water for a couple minutes on low. Add 1-3 cinnamon sticks, ginger root, and blend for 2 more minutes until smooth. Pour in GLASS or WOOD for storage. When plastic is heated, it releases chemicals. Store in refrigerator for up to 10 days.

- You can drink the gel straight up or add it to a nice smoothie.

- One of our favorite smoothies has 3oz of Irish moss gel, 1 banana, a handful of spinach, a teaspoon of vanilla, 10oz hemp or almond milk, and 4 dates. Make your own combinations, maybe add flaxseed or chia seed. Have fun with it.

- A few more herbs that are big in Jamaica are Guinea hen weed and Black Seed. Big Shirley swears by this stuff! They treat so many dis-eases such as, cancer, bacteria, virus infections, muscle spasms, fevers, regulates blood sugar/pressure, anti-inflammatory, and relax nerves.

- Cerasee tea – is also a bitter herb that is excellent for diabetes, high blood pressure, colds, liver repair, and constipation.

NEEK'S GENERAL RULES:

For starters eat: 50% raw food (organic uncooked fruits and vegetables) and 50% cooked foods

For the veterans: 70% raw foods, 30% steamed foods (may increase during winter months)

For sufferers from dis-ease:100% Raw/live foods for 12-18 weeks (maybe more).

For everyone: Avoid fried foods, frozen foods, salted foods. Refined, preserved foods, coffee, soda, alcohol, unnatural juice, white flour, white rice, and white sugar.

Fast in the beginning of the month at least 24 hours to reset your digestive system.

Steady treatments I live by aside from clean eating are:

- Acupuncture and Deep tissue massage

- Sauna/steam for 15 minutes

- Epsom salt bath soak for 20 minutes

- Enemas (coffee or warm water with cascara sagrada)

- Yoga and meditation

**Don't forget to burn some Sage to
"bun out di bad mind people dem"**

Final Thoughts and Take Away Points:

As Dr. Sebi says, "There is said to be one disease, the blood disease." Our blood is dependent on three things: What we think, what we eat, and what we inhale. To have optimal health is to have control over all three. We have little to no control over the air we breathe, which is typically worst in the inner cities. But in the matter of eating and drinking, we have conscious and deliberate control. By right eating, we may be healthy, even if we have not learned to control our thoughts. My plan in this book is to tackle diet and thought; you're on your own with the air.

Healing is not only faith-based. I know plenty of so-called "heathens" in great shape with good physical health. What goes on in their minds is a different story. You can pray for deliverance from disease, but if you continue wrong habits that go against nature, you will most likely remain dis-eased.

Our Kemetic (African Egyptian) Ancestors taught us that there are seven doctors of nature: Air *Water *Sunlight *Meditation *Food *Exercise *Fasting. Here are a few things to keep in mind:

- As soon as you wake up have a glass of filtered water (8oz) room temperature or warm water with lemon to activate your digestive system and clear out the nightly mucus build-up and toxins

- Eat from 12pm-7pm

- Break your fast (breakfast) with fresh organic fruits

- Drink green vegetable juices two times a day if possible

- Take a bath or shower everyday (can add sea salt to bath)

- Allow at least twenty minutes for digestion of fruits before eating any other food

- Go out into nature daily and get some fresh air and sun

- Get at least seven hours of sleep

- Add powdered spirulina supplement to smoothies/juice for a rich source of protein

- Eat a cooked lunch and a raw dinner

- IF IT'S WHITE, DON'T EAT IT

- If possible, only buy organic

- Our heaviest meal should be lunch (between 1pm-3pm)

- Fruits and animal protein combined ferment in the stomach causing indigestion, heartburn and gas

- Animal protein digests in the stomach producing uric acid. When sugars from starch are ingested simultaneously it creates more acid; leading to indigestion, heartburn and gas.

- Supplements should be organic and preferably from vegetarian sources

- Snacking prevents the body from going through a detoxification process; putting food on top of last night's undigested food acidifies the body causing inflammation

- Do not eat late at night because your metabolism is not working effectively to break down food well. When you eat late, you're stepping on the gas to cell degeneration which leads to aging.

- The most important sleep takes place from approximately 10pm-2am.

- I would suggest your last meal to be consumed at least three hours prior to bed

- Get annual physicals

- Cook with stainless steel, cast iron, ceramic, and glass bakeware

We need visualization to keep the motivation. Focus on your motivation – state the change you want to see in your life, and write it down with the outcome you desire. Set a realistic plan with a time frame. Don't make drastic changes; be patient with your body and trust the process.

Now practice your new habits and remember, a positive attitude is extremely important in restoring health!

---

33. Hartfield, Will. 7 Powerful Ways To Stimulate Hair Growth January 9th, 2019. Htttps://www.hairlossrevolution.com/how-to-stimulate-new-hair-growth/

PART II:
"KNOW THYSELF"

—AFRICAN PROVERB

In this next section, I will uncover lies taught and things omitted in our educational system. I have a vast appreciation for history and truly believe that in order for us to heal ourselves physically, we have to be aware of what has been fed to us psychologically. There is a deep connection between the foods you ingest, the thoughts in your mind that lead to the words you eject, and the spiritual awakening of people of color. What you have ingested mentally is the reason for what you are ingesting physically today.

I start the next section with a powerful quote from Malcolm X, who was well aware of the brainwashing being done to our people. This section is extremely important for overall well- being. I know you will enjoy it

"We are off our diet because we are off our culture"

—DR. LAILA AFRIKA

16

THE LIES MY TEACHER TOLD ME

"Little innocent black children, born of parents who believed
their race had no history. Little black children seeing, before they
could talk, that their parents considered themselves inferior.
Innocent black children growing up, living out their lives, dying
of old age-and all of their lives ashamed of being black."

−MALCOLM X

We are introducing a section on history here in order to begin eliminating the slave mindset from how we have been educated, which is intertwined with our slave eating habits. You will understand the link between the two subjects as you read along. Enjoy.

There is a grave mistrust between people of color and the medical, religious, political, law enforcement, and educational system in America. The first issue – which is what we come into contact with from sometimes three years old all the way up until seventeen years old – is the Department of Education School System.

From the moment they step into a classroom, the indoctrination of American history upon our children of color begins. The reason I mention only children of color is because two things are happening when a black/brown child and a white child are sitting in a classroom under instruction. A white child is being educated on how their people have saved the dull minded black race and have further advanced civilization. Meanwhile, the black child is learning that they were nothing more than slaves that had no culture, no spirituality, and are an uncivilized race.

There is a sense of pride/arrogance running through the veins of one child and a sense of inferiority/inadequacy in the other. One of the most pivotal times in history taught to all children in America turned into a mockery was the "discovery of America." Clearly, we are not slaves (in the physical sense) right now, but as Dr. Joy Degruy says, we are suffering from what is known as "Post Traumatic Slave Syndrome."

CHRISTOPHER "KILL"UMBUS

The Christopher Columbus account of his experience is everything but the truth, and the educational system insists on regurgitating this lie throughout our entire school experience. Columbus is portrayed virtually as an "American war hero," when he was nothing short of an uneducated murderer, who is honored yearly on a national holiday. When I reflect back on the myths learned about Columbus on his voyage, it further strengthens the argument that this system is not broken; it's just not for people of color.

Do you think the Department of Education is unaware of the lies our teachers have taught us, and now our children? We must pay attention to what our textbooks are telling us and what they are not telling us. What we read in our books today is a heroic adventure. There is no bloodshed – and just like that "Happy Columbus Day."

History in America is just that – HIS-STORY. Not our story, so we have to teach our youths and even adults who aren't aware of the atrocities that ultimately led to our demise. If we don't know who we were prior to slavery, we won't understand why it is imperative to reverse the psychological damage done to our people. This is one of the reasons we continue to obstruct our bodies and continue to eat like slaves. It is also the reason we continue to seek validation with our money, cars, clothes, and even partners; rather than seek higher consciousness through cleansing and respecting our bodies.

"They started without food in our mouth
They gave us pork and pig intestines
Shit you discarded that we ingested"

−JAY Z

We ingest all kinds of meats, sweets, fried foods, soda, alcohol, and drugs on a daily basis, further damaging our mind, body and soul. Mental growth is needed in order to solve our issues. A dynamic change can be sought after, once we stop voluntarily damaging our brain and nervous system with what we eat and how we think. Unfortunately, a lot of what and how we think is based on what we learned in school and how we were raised at home.

"There is a clear indication of deception between Christopher Columbus and his pilots. If he originally set out to go to the East Indies, why did he go to the West Indies? This is why the indigenous people, the Caribs and the Arawak's, are referred to as Indians."[61]

Columbus anticipated that the world was much smaller. One fourth of the way on his journey, he came across "the Americas," where he was met by the Arawak Americans who were very gentle and had rich culture (Arawak's were also referred to as Taino-Arawak.) The first slaves were not Africans, but Native Americans.

He then sailed to Cuba and Hispaniola (now Haiti and Dominican Republic.) He didn't find as much gold as he was looking for, but it was enough for him to have the Arawak's on Hispaniola mine gold for them, prepare food and reward his lieutenants with native women to rape.

Haitian people were not present-day Haitians as you imagine them. The native people on that island were Arawak's who were decimated by the mid-16th century. In 1495, Columbus rounded up 1500 Arawak men, women, and children for voyage back to Spain to be sold in order to pay back dividends to those who financed his expedition. Of the five hundred, two hundred died in route from diseases (such as small pox) from the Europeans. The island people had no natural immunity to that disease or other viruses carried by their conquerors.

MURDER FOR PROGRESS

All of Columbus's expeditions were financed by Spain's King Ferdinand and Queen Isabella, so he knew he had to come back with gold in order to pay back dividends to his investors. Columbus made a promise to fill the ships with gold, but when it became clear that there was no gold left, he had to take them as slaves. The Arawak's attempt to defend themselves failed, so they were taken as slave labor on their land. When Spaniards enslaved them, they were sometimes hung, burned to death, or the Arawak's killed themselves and their infants.

"In two years, through murder, mutilation, or suicide, half of the 250,000 Indians on Haiti were dead."[62] The Arawak's that remained through slave labor continued dying off by the thousands due to harsh labor conditions, murder, or disease. "By 1515, there were perhaps fifty thousand Indians left. By 1550, there were five hundred. A report of the year 1650 shows none of the original Arawak's or their descendants left on the islands." [63]

Columbus and his followers did not arrive on desolate land. They were met there with indigenous people who already had a culture far more extensive than theirs. They were densely populated and were more democratic than those in Europe. The only thing in which Arawak's were inferior to Europeans was their military capabilities. Once the entire native population was decimated, the next means to continue "advancing" the Americas and the surrounding Caribbean islands was to enslave Africans.

Slavery existed in African countries, and that fact is sometimes used by Europeans to justify the slave trade. Much like the serfs in Europe, Africa had similar practices where a slave might marry, own a slave, or property. Most people who became slaves became so as a product of war. Two different societies went to war for whatever reason and the loser became the slave. Slavery in Africa by African people was nothing like what the Trans-Atlantic Slave trade did to black people, who were considered personal property for 246 years.

FROM ARAWAK'S TO AFRICANS

Slavery of the African people in America has crippled our community, destroyed families, and stripped us of our spiritual practices. When indigenous people refer to the spirit, they are talking about the life force in everything. Spirit is deeply filled within the indigenous community. Community is the spirit whereby people come together to fulfill their purpose. When you don't have a community, you feel empty; like you don't belong and have no one to listen to you. You have no affirmation of who you are, which disempowers your psyche, making you helpless when removed from that type of environment.

This is the prime reason why families were torn apart, the men were emasculated in front of the women, and foreign religions were forced on the slaves. Slavery has disconnected us so much that we are terrified of our African ancestors' traditions and spiritual practices.

Before we continue with the lies taught in school, I want to first add an excerpt from the Willie Lynch Letter so we can better understand the minds of colonizers. In the 1700's this is the letter that was read to the white slave owners to teach them how to "break the Negro."

"Therefore, if you break the female, she will break the offspring in its early years of development and, when the offspring is old enough to work, she will deliver it up to you for her normal female protective tendencies will have been lost in the original breaking process...

Take the meanest and most restless nigger, strip him of his clothes in front the remaining niggers, the female, and the nigger infant, tar and feather him, tie each leg to a different horse faced in opposite directions, set him afire and beat both horses to pull him apart in front of the remaining niggers. The next step is to take a bullwhip and beat the remaining nigger male to the point of death in front of the female and the infant. Don't kill him...

By her being left alone, unprotected, with male image destroyed, the ordeal caused her to move from the psychological dependent state to a frozen independent state. In this frozen psychological state of independence, she will raise her male and female offspring in reverse roles. For fear of the young male's life, she will psychologically train him to be mentally weak and dependent but physically strong.[64] (The Willie Lynch Letter and The Making of a Slave)

- Can you agree that the effects of slavery referred to in this letter are happening right now?

- Can you agree that a lot of women of color seem to have an over-bearing independency issue, sometimes not allowing us to let a man lead the family? Are most women of color more comfortable supporting their man with his dreams or would they prefer him work for a corporation because it is "safe?"

- Can you agree that a lot of men of color are very dependent upon their mothers and are mentally weak?

IM NOT BLACK, I'M SPANISH

For the purpose of reframing the mindset we have had towards the country of Ayiti (Haiti), my focus will remain on this country, as opposed to the other enslaved countries of Jamaica, Trinidad, Bahamas, Puerto Rico, Guyana, Cuba etc. This country was the first to be emancipated and is the most connected to the original practices of our ancestors and is now demonized for it. The worst part is the most demonizing comes from our own people due to their ignorance of the Haitian Revolution.

After wiping out the Arawak people and replacing them with African people, slavery reached new heights in Hispaniola. The French and Spanish divided the island amongst themselves in the Treaty of Ryswick of 1696. Saint-Domingue in the west and Santo Domingo in the east. On the island during the late 1700's, there were white land owners, the mixed race "colored people" (descendants of the white owners and slaves), and the African slaves. Mixed race persons did not want to be associated with being African, but they weren't white enough to have equal privilege as land owners. This left them in a very uncomfortable position. The skin color differences became defining characteristics of what is now Haiti and Dominican Republic for the rest of history, or at least until we change history.

Eventually the ratio of white, mixed, and African changed drastically. The white land owners found themselves outnumbered which led to multiple slave rebellions. Africans who escaped from slavery and established free communities in mountainous regions were called "Maroons." These Maroons held on to their heritage of communal society and would run away in groups to re-establish villages. Maroons also spearheaded massive rebellions, such as Francois Makandal's, between 1751 and 1757.

"Makandal's most feared method of killing plantation owners was to instruct slaves to administer various plant poisons to their food, to blow poisonous powders in their faces, or to scatter poisons where they might walk barefoot or otherwise touch them."[65]

Vodou is also science. We also have another Maroon leader (Boukman, a Vodou priest) from Jamaica who is well known for freeing slaves during the Haitian revolution. Why were there Jamaicans in Haiti during the revolution? Because they understood that before being Jamaican, they were African first. Jamaicans are Haitians and Haitians are Jamaicans. During 1792, over one hundred plantations were burned to the ground and approximately four thousand slave owners were killed, allowing the rebels to control more than one third of Saint-Domingue.

In addition to the slave revolts, the French encountered another issue. The Spanish portion of the island (Santo Domingo), linked up with the British in attempting to invade and take over Saint-Domingue. Why? While all the slave revolts were happening, naturally France began to panic and reached out to the mixed race class and the white class for assistance in putting a stop to the slave rebellions. The conversation went a little something like this:

> **France:** "Hey white people, do you mind joining forces with the lighter black people so we can put a stop to these niggers killing slave owners? By the way, I plan to give them the same rights as you guys."

White people: "Ummm, what kind of crack are you smoking?"

France declared the colored people full citizens and granted them the same rights as white people. This move backfired on France because the white people did not consider light-skinned people white, and had no interest in being associated with them on any level. So what did the white class do? They called Great Britain to come save them from these crazy ass French people and requested to make Saint-Domingue a British colony instead.

Ultimately, the French gave Africans their freedom, supplied them with arms, and they joined together in battle in order to drive the Spanish and British out of the colony. The British rolled up in Saint-Domingue in heavy numbers, and the white land owners in the country were hoping they would reinstate slavery and strip the colored people of their citizen title and equal rights. The war between the British and the French started in 1794 and ended in 1801 with the French successfully driving the British and Spanish out of the colony. On January 3, 1801, all the people on the island of Hispaniola were freed. This was the first emancipation in the Western Hemisphere.

More specifically, Haiti was the world's first black republic born on January 1, 1804. Jean-Jacques Dessalines was elected governor and stood firm that no slave owner would ever control Haiti again. Something pivotal occurred during Dessalines' reign that would shape hostile race relations on the island of Hispaniola for decades.

"Dessalines' decision to declare all people equal and reduce Haiti's number of classes to one was well received-except amongst the country's remaining *gens de couleur*, who still chafed at the idea of being equated with Africans. Despite all of Dessalines's efforts to break the skin-color castes of Saint-Domingue and finally unite its multicultural people, subtle and blatant hostility and discrimination between light-skinned and dark-skinned Haitians continues into the current day, although it has no legal backing. In 1806, when Haiti's predominantly lighter skinned south rose up in revolt against its darker-skinned north, instead of supporting their leader, Dessalines's mixed-race generals had him murdered on his way to battle."[66]

WHY IS HAITI IN DEBT TO FRANCE?

Fast forward to when Haiti and Spanish Haiti were controlled by President Boyer from 1822 to 1843. "In 1825, France offered to recognize Boyer's government and Haiti as a legitimate and independent country - but only if Haiti was willing to pay for the privilege, with a massive sum of 150 million francs (equivalent to $21.7 billion in current U.S. dollars) to be paid over five years. Perhaps because the offer was delivered by a dozen French warships with their hundreds of cannons pointed at Haiti's capital, or perhaps for some other reason, Boyer signed the agreement."[67]

You can see how this can destroy a country's economy and start a never-ending cycle of international debt. According to present day Europeans, Haiti is in the situation it is in because they used voudou and the island is now cursed. Ridiculous! Haiti's only curse has been the European colonizers and corrupt politicians. Dessalines, Christophe, and L'Ouverture were great political rulers of Haiti and to their misfortune, died miserably because of their love for the country. Dessalines was assassinated by the same people he was trying to help. Christophe was driven to suicide, and L'Ouverture was set up and died in prison.

Ultimately, Spanish Haiti (now called the Dominican Republic) and French Haiti would remain divided. What I gave you is a short version of the history of Hispaniola, so we can all admire the strength of that country and its people, which are our people. We are the same and must treat each other as such.

If you are interested in more on this topic, I want you to research Rafael Trujillo to see how deep the hatred runs amongst our people because of the varying hues of our skin. The division between light-skinned and dark-skinned people is something we see happening with people of the United States and all around the world today. Dark-skinned men wanting children with lighter skinned women and vice versa – afraid of their children being born with too much melanin. In order to love one another and regain strength in our community, we have to stop hating ourselves. White man knew cross-breeding themselves with Africans would put us in this disgusting situation.

"Cross-breeding niggers means taking drops of good white blood and putting them into as many nigger women as possible, varying the drops by the various tones that you want, and then letting them breed with each other until the circle of colors appear as you desire… Cross-breeding completed, for further severance from their original beginning, we must completely annihilate the mother tongue of both the nigger and the new mule and institute a new language that involve the new life's work of both. You know, language is a peculiar institution. It leads to the heart of the people."[67]

They made you afraid to go to a country where we have the most attachment to our ancestors, but they are going there in numbers. Mainly to learn of voudou because they know that their major western religions – Islam, Judaism and Christianity – are all based on foundations from indigenous, African spiritual systems. They took this spiritual system, went back home and reinterpreted it to their people as their primary path to salvation.

For instance, King Solomon who lived from 976-936 B.C.E wrote what is known to you in the Bible as the "proverbs of King Solomon of Israel." Comparatively, we have Pharaoh Amenenope, who lived from 1405-1370 B.C.E., who wrote, "The Teachings of Amenemope." He lived more than three hundred years before King Solomon, but if you view both of their works, they're almost exactly the same. This is just one of many examples of "coincidences" you find throughout history. Research it for yourself; don't just take my word for it.

Now I'm not saying to give up on your current religion of choice. I'm saying show respect to where it came from. Don't look down on our brothers and sisters from Haiti, Africa or any other culture, and presume that they or the country are evil because they practice voudou or something you don't understand.

Haitian voudou is a spiritual practice and a way of life. It's not just filled with magic and murder; these views were a huge part of the European propaganda to further sever ties from our culture. Have you noticed that all non-white cultures or spirituality are branded as pagan, ungodly, heathen-like? Whenever two cultures/countries reach the final face off, the dominant ruler will take whatever is beneficial or positive to add to their culture and leave the rest to be branded as wicked, evil, or ungodly. Has the oppressor ever taught the oppressed anything that can have them move forward as a strong people?

Can evil happen in voudou? Yes, but you are responsible for all consequences that come with it. Some may call this "karma." Voudou has helped people heal themselves of sicknesses, mental disturbances, and spiritual imbalances. Overall, I am saying that voudou is not evil, the evil is in the heart. A number of separate cultural influences from Africa and the indigenous Taino on Hispaniola merged together to create Haitian Voudou. If you learn about it from an actual Voudou priest, you will understand it better and may even deem it to be beautiful.

I came to a crossroad in my life where I questioned a lot in the religion I was in at the time. A lot of things weren't making sense to me. Questions couldn't be answered, and I was left to just have faith, but it was too late; I had to know more. From around 2008, even up until now, I was led on a life-long journey of searching and searching to find the truth…my truth. When I was seeking something of traditional heritage, in a divine way, I was brought back to the spiritual practices of my ancient ancestors in Africa. My goal now is to continue to pass through stages of conscious development until I reach the highest level.

Everything is in reverse now in America. What do I mean? A great number of Caucasian people eat healthy, support each other, and practice yoga, meditation, and spirituality. A great number of Africans in America eat terrible, practice religion, don't exercise, and support everyone but their own. This is not how it was pre-slavery. We need to get back to our culture.

"Until Haiti spoke… no Christian nation had abolished slavery. Until she spoke… the slave trade was sanctioned by all the Christian nations of the world… Until Haiti spoke, the church was silent and the pulpit dumb."

−FREDRICK DOUGLAS, 1893

Research the history of your people and do not leave it to school to give you knowledge of self, or you will go through your entire life not understanding the true meaning of who you are and why you are here. Ingest the truth and teach your children the truth.

"You have to be careful, very careful, introducing the truth to black man who has never previously heard the truth about himself, how own kind, and the white man."

−MALCOLM X

61. John Henrik Clarke. *Christopher Columbus and the Afrikan Holocaust*; Slavery and the Rise of Ruropean Capitalism. Published by Eworld Inc., Buffalo, New York (1998), pg.48.

62. Zinn, Howard. *A Peoples History of the United States*, Harper Perennial Modern Classics, New York, New York, (2005), pg. 5.

63. *The Willie Lynch Letter and the Making of a Slave*, African Tree Press, pg. 5.

64. Mambo Chita Tann. *Haitian Vodou, An Introduction to Haiti's Indigenous Spiritual Tradition*. Llewellyn Publications Woodbury, Minnesota, (2016), pg. 23.

65. Mambo Chita Tann. *Haitian Vodou. An Introduction to Haiti's Indigenous Spiritual Tradition*. Llewellyn Publications Woodbury, Minnesota, (2016), pg. 29.

66. Mambo Chita Tann. *Haitian Vodou. An Introduction to Haiti's Indigenous Spiritual Tradition*. Llewellyn Publications Woodbury, Minnesota (2016), pg. 31.

67. *The Willie Lynch Letter and the Making of a Slave*, African Tree Press pg. 23-25.

17

EDUCATION AND MEDICATION

This miseducation of our people has led me to address issues with our youth. It is quite apparent that America unequivocally associates black children with special Ed, therefore killing their dreams before they grow-up. It begins like this this…

"Ms. Samuels, your child is too hyper."

"Ms. Samuels, your child is unable to sit still."

"Ms. Samuels, I think your child has some behavioral issue."

These words sound all too familiar to families of color. Being called into school to sit down with your child's teacher, the school psychologist and maybe even the principal. "Ms. Samuels, we think Safaree may have a behavioral issue and we would like to have him tested."

Typically, a lot of parents would agree to testing because let's face it – these adults have degrees so they must be right. Right? HELL NO! Not in all the cases that have come about. Luckily for my brother, my mom said no to testing, let alone medication. Fast forward, thirty years later and he is living out his dreams, drug free.

If you think it's absolutely normal to have a child confined to a chair for seven hours with a one-hour lunch break and sit straight through it without agitation, it's not. I can barely do that myself. Our ancestors did not educate us in a room for several hours; we were educated outside. We are sunlight dependent people whose brains are stimulated by light. The intelligence is dulled because the electromagnetic circuitry needed to stimulate our cells to communicate to one another is decreased due to lack of light. Manipulate the light, manipulate the brain.

We need to get away from unnatural light, radiation (microwaves, computers, televisions, videogames, cell phones) and get into nature, get into the sun.

My daughter is going to an amazing preschool called "The Little Sun People." They didn't choose this name by accident. This is a school that focuses on black greatness, and the history of our movement.

Ultraviolet radiation exposure on melanin-dominate people has a negative effect on our thinking capabilities. What does this mean? Don't allow the television or video games to raise your children. Don't allow teachers, counselors, and a few degrees intimidate you into going along with any recommendations.

The system loves to throw around the term "learning disability." We all have a learning disability. My ability to learn may not be the same as your ability to learn. Maybe I'm better at math in the morning, and you're better in the afternoon. In a learning structure, we are all very different and learn differently. This needs to be nourished, not demonized. We need to take time to evaluate where this information is coming from. We have excellent teachers, but we also have teachers that don't have the patience for normal child-like behavior. Some of these teachers are part of "the system" we spoke of earlier to keep us in the position that we are in and have been in far too long.

TOO BLACK & TOO NAPPY

Watching a lecture by Dr. Jewel Pookrum taught me something I think is absolutely remarkable. Our community has a huge issue with embracing blackness. Due to racial inequalities and self-image, we try to bleach our skin, hide from the sun, not interact with too many black people etc…

The hate you have for yourself creates a chemical reaction in your brain. I will summarize this portion of Dr. Pookrum's lecture as such: Individuals that have issues with melanin, because they are not able to utilize the molecule openly and receptively, their thoughts create chemicals from the brain that actually deactivate the molecule.

"Your brain attacks the aspect of yourself that you are having issues with and will render that aspect inactive or bring about its destruction. Self-hate can lead to deactivation of your melanin molecules which will bring about dis-ease. Your thoughts can disable your ability to function."[68]

In laymen's terms, if you hate yourself your body cells will attack you. I find that so fascinating because this is something we have to instill in our young children who are constantly being told directly or indirectly that they need to be white or that our race is inferior. It's such an early age to begin self-destruction leading up until adulthood.

Melanin is an intricate part of your being. Your perception of what you know about it and how you use it can allow you to have total access to anything in the universe, or it can be responsible for you creating your own demise. That is so powerful.

MURDER BY PRESCRIPTION

Let's say my mother did agree to behavioral testing for my brother. Here comes our friends from the medical monopoly to offer you Prozac, Ritalin, or any drug used to treat Attention Deficit Disorder or any type of behavioral condition. Now, we have started a cycle with a six or seven year-old boy who now believes he must take drugs to function in society. That's a real confidence builder to go along with the history lessons that you are nothing, came from nothing, and will never be nothing.

And yes, there are children who may learn a bit slower than what we are accustomed to, but my suggestion is to give them more one-on-one time before you opt to medicate them. There is a huge target on colored children, especially boys. It is no coincidence that more men of color are in prison, special education classes, unemployed, raised in single parent households…etc.

Now raise your hand if you are waiting for things to improve naturally.

If you raised your hand, please go back to the beginning of this book and start again. That kind of thinking lacks critical reasoning. Before agreeing to medication, first check your child's diet. Is it filled with flesh foods and sugar which produces similar effects on the brain as cocaine?

Scientist have shown that sugar has an addictive power similar to illegal drugs which can cause cravings, depression, hyperactivity, ADHD, binges and withdrawal symptoms. Brain imaging showed excess sugar increased slow brain waves. A sugary diet contributes to lack of focus and attention. When we eliminate or reduce our children's sugar intake, they will have a greater ability to focus. They will continue to strengthen their natural ability to be independent entrepreneurs. We have continuously added to the forward movement of other people's cultures and need to have the next generation add to ours. Teach your children to become producers, not consumers.

It is not impossible to get children to eat healthy, as one would presume. For myself, I started my daughter Melia a certain way from birth. At five years old, she has never had McDonalds, KFC, Wendy's, or even cow's milk. Sun people need citrus fruits – lemon, lime, grapefruit, and oranges. These are known to have a lot of hydrogen like the sun. Our children also need water, not massive amounts of juice. These things will assist greatly with their cognitive function. For those of us who have to transition our child off a diet high in sugar and junk, we can do it slowly. I found that when I allow my child to prepare her own smoothies, juices or small meals, she is more inclined to try them.

Carrots and beets are high in natural sugar, so use them moderately when preparing juices. Rule of thumb is to try not to exceed 25% of your juicing with these two vegetables and don't let the juice sit; drink it right away. Kids want to be healthy and they want to do well in school. What child says, "Hey mom and dad, I want to fail in school, have all my peers hate me, and don't forget to load me up with poisons so I can time my speedy death?" None!

Kids follow what people do more than what they say so it starts with us. When adults resist something, it's not because they don't believe it will work; it is more so a fear of change. Your thinking is your only limitation in this life. Our children are not born with a desire to destroy their lives, let alone their bodies. They are taught to connect McDonald's with pleasure and vegetables with punishment. Their little bodies need a strong nutritional foundation to prepare them for the future.

We have a lot of work to do, so let's make sure our children, family, friends, and more importantly ourselves are properly hydrated, nourished, deeply loved and spiritually connected in order embark on our journey as what we used to be, a community.

In ancient Kemet (today known as Egypt) above the entrance of each temple is inscribed, "KNOW THYSELF." This thought is commonly attributed to Socrates the Greek, but our African ancestors created this philosophical statement which is pivotal in this time. More than ever before, our children need to have knowledge of self, and until we create our own schools, it must start at home.

Every direction a child of color turns, there are huge signs telling them they need to be white. This can lead to them rejecting the image they see in the mirror. Let's take action with simple steps. Talk to your child every day. Ask them about what they did in school or ask more specific question so that you don't get short three-word answers like, "I learned today."

Don't just buy them what you never had, teach them what you never knew. We all need to listen to our children more and not allow the television or any type of media to raise them. Imagery is extremely strong, especially when dealing with the youth's sponge-like brains.

I have a Bachelor's Degree in Graphic Design and learned the science, down to colors of images and their power on the mental. You hear and see the garbage that flows through our electronic devices. Do you know who runs the media? The same medical monopoly trying to provide you or your child with prescriptions that have 100 or more side effects.

> **"Everyman teaches as he acts. He will speak to the children so that they will speak to their children."**
>
> −AFRICAN PROVERB

HYERACTIVITY REMEDY:

ADD (ADHD)/HYPERACTIVITY is an imbalance in the brain that can be treated with natural remedies along with a CHANGE IN DIET. To assist with removal of pesticides, mercury, lead, artificial sweeteners, white sugar, antibiotics, processed foods etc. we would introduce:

- St. John's Wort – calms the nervous system and is the herb of choice for children

- Valerian – reduces restlessness and improves sleep

- Grapeseed Extract – protects the brain against a wide variety of poisons and improves blood flow.

- Ginkgo – fights free radicals and improves circulation to brain. Stimulates pineal gland to produce melanin. Alcohol free tincture of 8 drops 1-3X a day.

- Echinacea & Goldenseal – a natural immune booster.

- Vitamins & Minerals – vitamins E, C and B - complex, magnesium, calcium, zinc.

Sample tincture combination: 1tsp of Ginkgo, 1tsp of St. John's Wort, 1tsp of Valerian, ¼ tsp of peppermint leave, 1tsp of catnip. Mix ingredients and give ½ dropper full 3-4 times a day.

-NO WHITE SUGAR, BROWN SUGAR, LIMIT SALT, NO ALCOHOL OR VINEGAR, NO CANDY, NO CEREAL, NO DAIRY, NO RED MEAT OR PORK, NO ARTIFICAL JUICES, NO FROZEN FOODS, NO CHOCOLATE, NO MICROWAVE USE AND NO FAST FOODS.

-Diet should include fresh fruits, green juices and vegetables. Natural toothpaste only.

-No fluorescent lights (frequency of this light induces hyperactivity) - Chroma or incandescent light bulbs are best.

-**Please be patient with the child**. They did not ask for ADHD, they are simply reacting to the effects of it.

VACCINE INGREDIENTS

I want to list the ingredients in vaccines that I learned from a lecture called "Journey Back to Health" by Dr. Laila O. Afrika. He received the ingredients from the *Black Star* paper, April Edition. I have my daughter in school, so of course she was vaccinated. I just spread them out instead of following the doctor's typical rules of injecting her month after month after month. This is extremely important to be aware of because I learned Japan banned immunization of infants under two years old. They understand that a newborn does not have his/her own immune system to respond to these toxic chemicals.

I truly believe that it is the over vaccinating that is causing development issues in our youth such as autism. The mercury, also labeled "thimerosal", added to vaccine is so toxic that if a mercury filled thermometer breaks on the floor, the entire building has to evacuate. For the entire allopathic medical system to embrace poisoning babies as the norm is pure madness. There are stories you can research yourself from parents across the globe who stated that their child was perfectly normal prior to being vaccinated, which I believe is greatly due to the mercury. My child does not get the flu shot because no one in my family or her dad's family has ever had the flu or the shot. As you have seen from references throughout the book FDA approval means absolutely nothing regarding safety. Here are a list of some of the ingredients, so you are aware of what is being injected into our little babies:

Aluminum, Pig, Horse, and Cattle Blood, Chick Embryo, Phenol, Benzehonium, Ethylene Glycol, Formaldehyde (embalming fluid), Gelatin, Thimerosol, Glutamate, Foreign Protein, Neomycin, Monkey or Dog Kidney, Animal RNA or DNA, Aborted Human Fetus Tissue, Rabbit Brain, Human Manure, Throat infectious Mucus, Proviruses, Trypsin (Pigs stomach), Cowpox Pus, Radiation, and Antibiotics.[69]

GUNS & BUTTER

One of the most important things that should be taught in school are finance, credit maintenance/building, and saving (financial education.) Not one class taught me any of these things growing up and most of us, unfortunately, had to learn the hard way. Over 300 years of slavery guaranteed European people from then until now privilege and prosperity, while some Africans suffer, from then until now, with debt and bad money management.

In the early 2000's, there was a vendor outside of my high school distributing credit card applications offering credit cards with limits from $500-$2000. Due to our brothers and sisters' lack of understanding regarding credit, we all applied for the cards, were approved and ultimately went on a shopping spree. What did they think we were going to do? Be responsible and pay our debt monthly? Hell no! We bought Iceberg, Moschino, Polo, and Coogi. Some of us actually thought it was free money. We have to teach our children about checks and balances; or like Melvin from the movie, *Baby Boy,* describes, "Guns and Butter."

Guns: Real Estate, Stocks and Bonds

Butter: Cars, Clothes and Jewelry

Quick personal story regarding my first experience with "Guns and Butter." I had excellent credit right out of high school and by age twenty-five, I went and bought my first gun. Not a real gun silly. I'm talking about a house. Don't congratulate me yet. My mind was still focused on butter and I made terrible decisions, which led to my eight-year demise of the bad credit debacle.

Long story short, I made a bad real estate investment at the worst possible time (2007 market crash.) The goal was to flip the house, make some quick money and buy "hot whips." I got stuck with the house. I didn't visit the house for years so I decided one day to visit with my friends Byrde and Ray. When we got there we found out the house was being rented out by my broker behind my back for years! That was short lived because raccoons ate through the roof and also became my tenants. The raccoons led the squatters to move out.

Fast forward to 2014, I sold the house for 1/8th of what I purchased it for and had bad credit for an additional 1.5 years. Although I understood the concept of savings, credit and investments, I still had that itch to make quick money, make it rain, and buy things that glitter. Like the old saying goes, "everything that glitters isn't gold." Moral of the story: Explain to our youths the difference between needs and wants. Not for nothing though; experience is a great teacher and I'll never do that again!

FINAL THOUGHT:

Children are natural born entrepreneurs. Unlike the conventional structure of education, we need to nourish that and continue to teach them principles of entrepreneurship. How can we find each child's super power through learning and build on it? Let's face it, most of us will have to work a "9-5" to finance our dreams for a little while, but America's goal is to kill that dream and have you working for their corporation for the rest of your life instead.

As a parent, I noticed something black parents do that is detrimental to their child before they are even born. We say, "I'm going to give my son a white person's name so that when they apply for a job and their resume is viewed, they will get a call back."

That's the most illogical thing I've ever heard because guess what? You still have to show up for the interview and unless you plan on bleaching your skin, you can't hide that you're black/brown. Before your child is born, you're planning for them to work a 9-5 instead of giving them a name that you truly want to give them that might have meaning.

Plan for them to not have to work for anyone. Start the work yourself so they can follow your lead into entrepreneurship and financial freedom. Typically it takes thirty to forty years before you can retire most jobs, and by that time, they're hoping you didn't take care of yourself, ate like shit those forty years, and will drop dead the moment you walk out of their doors.

"Whereas nature provides them with their natural capacity to take care of their needs and the needs of their offspring, we break that natural string of independence from them and thereby create a dependency state so that we may be able to get from them useful production for our business and pleasure."[70]

In the next chapter, we will touch on a few topics covering Our Story and not His-story that are seldom known or taught in our communities.

---

68. Pookrum, Jewel. Published March 24, 2016. Differences between Africans and other races and cell regeneration https://youtu.be/yJIF6BYS9po

69. Afrika, Laila O. Published October 17, 2016. Journey Back to Health. https://youtu.b/AWSi-SRZc78

70. *The Willie Lynch Letter and the Making of a Slave*, African Tree Press pg. 10.

18

BULLET PROOF MIND

"You must use knowledge given, otherwise it is useless. Many of the vibrations which seem negative are really from within our own self, not from outside conditions. Lack of mind balance often results in the arousing of such negative thoughts that we really feel as if outside entities or forces were at work on us."

-THE EMERALD TABLETS OF THOTH

TUSKEGEE SYPHILLIS EXPERIMENT

From 1932 to 1972 (forty years), there was a study being performed in Tuskegee, Alabama called, "Tuskegee Study of Untreated Syphilis in the Negro Male." This study was conducted by the U.S. Public Health Service in partnership with Tuskegee to track the progression of the deadly venereal disease, syphilis, without treatment. The participants were recruited with a promise of free medical care and had no idea they had syphilis. They were told they were being treated for "bad blood." The *Washington Star* newspaper broke this story in July of 1972.

In exchange for their participation, they were promised free medical exams, free meals, and a burial stipend. The men jumped at the chance because they were mostly impoverished, uneducated share-croppers who had never been to the doctor before. Six hundred black men – 399 were diagnosed with syphilis and 201 were a control group without the disease. The men with the disease were not told that they were, in fact, infected, and therefore were not treated. The worst part is a cure (penicillin) was discovered for syphilis in the late 1940's, but the health workers monitoring them only gave the men placeboes, such as aspirin and mineral supplements! Simply put, they were being watched until they died so their bodies could be examined for the ravages of the disease.

By the time Jean Heller blew the whistle on the story in the news-paper, 128 had died of syphilis itself or syphilis-related complications. When I think about this, my mind immediately tries to understand, why allow over one hundred men to die when you could have received the information you were looking for within the first one to five autop-sies at most?

The medical community watched them die to discover the effects of the disease in their bodies in comparison to a white person. I believe it has to do with the mysterious powerful effects of melanin in the body that are not available to the European community. This is a country that will advance medicine by any means necessary.

So how did this sad story end? With public outrage and a law-suit of course. The NAACP sued on behalf of the survivors and their infected families. The Federal Government settled for ten million dol-lars and free medical services. After going through that, who the hell would want their free medical services?!

Throughout American history, black people have been experi-mented on in the name of science. The syphilis experiment was going on up until 1972 and probably would have gone on longer if it wasn't for that one person who uncovered the story.

In the mid 1800's there was another physician, if you could even call him that, who frequently conducted surgical experiments on slaves. J. Marion Sims is credited with inventing the first vaginal speculum. Sims would regularly experiment on black women, with no anesthesia, because he asserted that black women were more durable due to their skin color. So many slaves died in Sim's "laboratory," but lucky for him, he could autopsy further into these interesting dark people.

He also experimented on infants, sometimes prying their skulls open with sharp objects such as a shoe maker awl, in an effort to fix their skull malformations. From the 1800's to 1972, we have concrete evidence of savagery committed by the medical community against our people of color.

Again, I go to the doctor every year, but I do not live my life carelessly. There are great people out there in medicine, but unfortunately, you don't know who you're going to get. Do not allow yourself to continue to be enslaved through diet and medicine.

THE BLACK WALL STREET
"From Promise Land to Waste Land"

The Red Summer of 1919 was a period where there was over twenty-five, anti-black riots in America between May and October. Whites were invading and destroying black communities due to racial strife sometimes aided by labor shortages. Police also assisted the white residents by attacking black businesses and homes. Many black soldiers returning home from WWI were outspoken against racial discrimination, violence and inequality that continued to plague black communities. After WWI, approximately 100,000 veterans moved north, where they continued to encounter harsh racism. The constant, unpunished lynching of black people by whites contributed to the KKK mentality, which fueled strong self-defense and unity among black people. It was called Red Summer because blood was literally flowing through the streets from the numerous deaths during the riots. Racial intolerance persisted throughout the States until 1921, where we had one of the worst riot/race wars in history.

In 1921, the racial intolerance spread like wildfire to Tulsa, Oklahoma. The population of the blacks totaled 11,000 out of almost 100,000 whites. The black people in this area were thriving immensely! They had two black public schools, a black hospital, banks, pharmacies, fraternal lodges, loan companies, real estate agents, barbers, fifteen physicians, dentists, surgeons, contractors, tailors, plumbers, restaurants, theaters, hotels, law firms and a multitude of productive businesses.

"White racism was a major impetus for growth of the Black Business District. Blacks could work in white areas as common laborers, domestics and in the service sector, but their money was not welcomed by white businesses... **The dollar circulated 36 -100 times, sometimes taking a year for currency to leave the community. Now a dollar leaves the black community in 15 minutes."**[71]

It is also noted that in this time, there were several black millionaires, some even owning private planes. If this community could make this happen in 1921, why can't we?

So what happened in Tulsa that would destroy what was called, "Little Africa?" A nineteen year-old black man named Dick Rowland was working in the Drexel building as a shoe shiner. He encountered an elevator operator named Sarah Page when he was heading to the restroom. When the elevator doors closed, she screamed and claimed she was assaulted. Dick Rowland was arrested; even though Page didn't formally press charges against him, the community did.

To add fuel to the fire, the *Tulsa Tribune* (major newspaper in town) wrote a story titled, "Nab Negro for Attacking Girl in Elevator." This inflammatory article strongly suggested that Rowland raped Page.

You know once that paper hit the streets, it was going down between black and whites! The white people gathered at the courthouse wanting Rowland lynched, but the black community came together and decided a lynching for an alleged assault was going too far. The African American community rushed to the courthouse, strapped with guns to protect Rowland.

While both communities were outside of the courthouse, a white man approached a black man with a gun and based on various accounts, asked him something like, "What are you gonna do with that gun nigger?" The black man answered, "Ima use it if I have to." The two men argued, a struggle over the gun ensued and a shot fired. The white resident was shot and all hell broke loose.

Blacks retreated back to the Greenwood District to set up a barrier to keep whites from entering their community. But because they were so outnumbered and outgunned, the white residents broke through the barriers. It was seventeen hours of anarchy, leaving Greenwood completely decimated without a building standing. Black residents' homes and businesses were looted and burned – approximately thirty-five city blocks. Police offers abandoned their duties to side with the white rioters. Black men were rounded up by the police and taken to detention centers, leaving the community defenseless. Reports have said that airplanes were involved in the riots, dropping nitro glycerin throughout the town, setting it ablaze.

So how did this all end? The National Guard had to get involved to stop this murder spree by declaring martial law. Approximately 300 people were killed. The blacks who survived were brought to internment centers temporarily, but once they returned home, they were living in tents. This case was brought to trial, but the State Grand Jury pretty much said that black people brought this on themselves. They did file charges against various people, but none of the cases were tried and no white person sent to prison.

Does any of this sound familiar in today's world? All insurance claims from the Greenwood neighborhood were DENIED, totaling a little over 2.7 million dollars. They never received any justice. Situations that happened in the 1800's are still happening til this day

BLACK PANTHERS

The Black Panthers was a pro-black organization created by Huey P. Newton and Bobby Seale. Their primary focus was to increase the rights of people of color through economic, political, medical, and educational advancement. When Malcolm X was assassinated on February 21st, 1965, Seale swore to pick up where Malcolm X left off.

The economic and political structure of black America was never challenged or changed with the voting act of 1965. Tensions were increasing as laws were being created, but there was no severe impact in the forward movement of the black community.

Most black families remained in poverty, living in the projects, going to overcrowded schools, and facing police brutality on a daily basis. This was a major speech driver of Malcolm X that resonated with the black community. There was no equal distribution of economic and political power to the black man in America who built this country for free.

Like today, most homicides were ruled justifiable and caused several rebellions to occur in Los Angeles. That eventually sparked community rage and the black people began looting, stealing guns, and shooting at helicopters and police offers.

To prevent further riots and rebellions, two brothers named Lennie and Crook organized CAP (Community Alert Patrol). CAP's purpose in organizing this patrol was to monitor police activity. Yes, monitor the police.

HAND OVER YOUR GUNS NIGGERS

Huey P. Newton studied law at Merritt College and San Francisco State College. There he discovered in California that you can carry loaded guns in public, as long as they were visible. Newton studied law inside out. "The Black Panther is an animal that when pressured, it moves back until it is cornered, then comes out fighting for life or death."[72]

Newton knew it was time for black people to unite and protect themselves and the community because the police, nor the government did. There was a situation where Newton and Seale were patrolling the police with their shot gun and M-1 in their laps. They pulled up next to some "pigs" (their words not mine) and the cops noticed the firearms and threw their lights on.

Newton ignored the lights and kept driving. Apparently, you have to have sirens as well. The cops then threw the sirens on and Seale and Newton pulled over. When the cops approached them, they demanded that the "niggers hand over their guns," but Newton and Seale refused and began citing their rights. After a lot of back and forth, the lieutenant arrived and told his officers that they couldn't arrest them because they were exercising their rights. This is one of many acts that sparked interest from the community about the Black Panther Party.

With black people now empowered with carrying arms, take a wild guess as to what happened next? Assemblyman at the time, Don Mulford, introduced a bill in the summer of 1967 making it illegal to carry firearms. Oh my God… I'm so surprised (sarcasm)!

That didn't stop the Panthers from fighting for basic human rights. Newton released a series of *Black Panther* newspapers, and in one of them, he expressed the black man's inferiority complex. "Many black men associated a sexual desire for white woman with a desire to be recognized as human and free."[73] He mentions how they blame themselves for their position or lack thereof, in society. The Black Panthers were doing what government, law enforcement, and the medical community would not – focus on the needs and interests in their community. They were not armed thugs looking for trouble. They were the voice of the people.

Newton also questioned the overuse of policing by police that weren't from the inner cities. Essentially, they felt that if the police had to come home to their neighborhoods to rest their heads at night, there would be less police brutality.

DOPE PROGRAMS

The Black Panthers did what authorities wouldn't do. They created programs for inner city kids, such as the "free breakfast for children program." They also provided free health clinics, a free clothes and shoes program, and youth programs. As mentioned in the Tuskegee Syphilis Experiment, most black people were poor and had never seen a doctor in their life. All clinics were run by volunteers who were nurses, interns, doctors, and medical students.

Drug addiction was a big problem in our community at this time so they also provided assistance in battling addiction. "The brothers build their program on the revolutionary ideology of capitalism plus dope equals genocide. **Dope, they argued, was part of the oppressors plan to ensure our enslavement.**"[74] What is interesting is that the drugs circulating in the black communities were provided by the CIA. The CIA admitted to smuggling drugs (mainly crack/cocaine) from Nicaragua into the inner city black neighborhoods in 1998.

One of the programs I absolutely loved was the free ambulance service. I can't imagine how long it must have taken for the EMT ambulance to arrive in the black/brown neighborhoods in the 60's! This amazing organization took matters into their own hands and did it themselves. "**Improving the health status of blacks, this went hand and hand with improving their political, economic, and social status.**"[75] They even created their own black empowerment education curriculum because similar to today, the department of education curriculum does not provide it. The Panthers were teaching us to build a nation for ourselves.

BLACK POWER=GOVERNMENT CORRUPTION

The government and the FBI strategically reversed the forward movement that the Black Panthers created. They found ways to stop businesses from supporting with food donations and program spaces. Their offices throughout America were being raided by police and members were being arrested, one being Afeni Shakur, Tupac Shakur's mother. The members were harassed, arrested, Panther offices tear gassed, and members sold each other out for less jail time. This would ultimately end the Black Panther Organization. Why put so much effort into destroying so-called weak, ignorant black people? Because they know more about you than you do. No one puts this much effort into destroying someone unless they are afraid of them.

> "**There will never be another black messiah unless we created him.**"
>
> – J. EDGAR HOOVER (FBI)

ANCIENT KEMET
Resurrection of our History and Culture

Typically, new information makes us uncomfortable and tends to lead us to reject it before ingesting it. For people hearing this information for this first time, it can be very overwhelming because it's not what we were taught in school. African spirituality focuses its teaching on learning about the universe, nature, and the mysteries of life. It strengthens our connection to our ancestors.

The name, Egypt, was imposed on ancient Kemetic people by foreigners. Let me first address what may seem to be basic knowledge, but is surprisingly not. Egypt is on the continent of Afraka or Alkebulan (now Africa.) There are people, sadly some Egyptologists that are trying to take Egypt out of Afraka.

Afraka literally means flesh and soul of the hidden sun. AF (flesh) Ka (soul) of the hidden Ra (sun.) A blind person can see that Egypt is not in the Middle East. You will see at the end of this section why Egypt is now an Arabic nation.

I'll be providing the information based on research by amazing African historians that have spent their lives researching ancient Kemet to provide us with the truth. Great thanks to Yosef A.A. ben-Jochannan, Ivan Van Sertima, John Henrik Clarke, Anthony T. Browder, George G.M. James, Queen Afua, and Cheikh Anta Diop.

There is a vast amount on information that came out of the Nile Valley from Kush (Ethiopia) to Kemet, so I want to give you a glimpse of our history prior to European and Arabic Invasion. Kush means "burnt or charred" and Kemet means "black land," which represents the people and rich dark soil along the Nile River. The Nile River is the only river that flows from south to north. It then empties into the Mediterranean Ocean. Ancient Kemetians have influenced civilization based on written records from 3100 B.C., and are the oldest recorded civilization on earth.

This is proven with the construction of Heru-em-akhet (Great Sphinx) monument on the Giza Plateau that dates back to 11,000 B.C. The original inhibitors of the Nile Valley unified to build this monument in honor of Sekhmet. The Kemetic (Egyptian) people were black and Egyptologists have put forth grand efforts in destroying a black Egypt at any and all cost.

Most pyramids were built on plateaus, showing you that they were the first civilization to have an irrigation system. The pyramids were acoustically tuned. They had running water and a sewer system. There is a constant denial to attribute black Africa's contribution to ancient civilization that influenced today's spiritual systems, astrology, biology, "Khem-mystery" (chemistry), anatomy, astronomy, art, Medu Neter (hieroglyphics), and the oldest calendar in existence. It is very difficult for Europeans to admit, let alone accept, that all these systems preceded Europe. Heck, most of us don't even believe it! For over a thousand years our perception of our race has been shaped by European colonizers and enslavers. True knowledge has been withheld so we would be subject to control by people who manipulate us through fear and ignorance.

Kemetians created books along with libraries. They are the creators of holistic living. Christianity, Judaism, and Islam are the offspring's of ancient Kemetic spiritual systems that foreigners learned while in Northern Egypt. They took what they learned back home and reinterpreted it in their own way to their own people as the road to deliverance.

They had their own system of law that the people followed called the 42 laws of MAAT. These laws represented peace, harmony, moral, justice and righteousness amongst the ancient people of Kemet and the divine cosmological order. Maat is designed to avert chaos and maintain truth. To learn more about the culture of Kemet, I highly recommend purchasing the oldest book in history, "Pert Em Heru" or *The Book of Coming Forth from Darkness into Light*. This book was erroneously labeled by Egyptologist as *The Book of the Dead* to keep you away from it.

Ancient Egypt had the first government that was ruled by monarchs and civil servants. Their system was based on spiritual values and they, for the most part, enjoyed an orderly society. They were not perfect, by any means, and had internal upheaval occur during certain periods throughout history, which eventually led to their demise. Ultimately, Egypt was weakened by the political, economic, and social turmoil's of war.

Maat is the reason the civilization was so great and lasted so long. Maat demanded accountability, which is something that is lacked in most religions. There is no "great judgment day" because every day is judgment day, and you are responsible for all of your actions.

Ancient Kemetics teach that we should eat when we are hungry and not out of habit. Eat to live and not live to eat. The saying "¼ of what you eat will keep you alive, the other ¾ will keep your doctor alive," comes from an issue that they experienced with overeating during ancient times. The way that they remedied this was to create a blueprint of what was best to eat and how much. Our ancestors spent millions of years perfecting what used to be our diet – fruits, vegetables, plant-based protein, natural grains, and once in a while, they ate meat. Our ancestors were not perfect by any means, but when there was an issue within the community, they worked hard to resolve it, not mask it.

ANIMAL WORSHIP? MULTIPLE GODS?

Contrary to popular belief, our ancient Kemetic ancestors were not pagans, polytheist, heathens, evil, or worshipping animals. Ancient Kemetians created and thought in terms of symbolism. It you take their teachings literal you will be confused and miss the entire point. They viewed "NTR" (Neter) as the Most High, creator of all things. NTR is comparable to the Christians' Jehovah. What Europeans mistakenly refer to as Gods and Goddesses were the characteristics/attributes of NTR. This is called an anthropomorphic representation of GOD.

For instance, the "god" Heru, who is known to most as Horus, represents your higher self. He is victory and who we call upon to overcome challenges and obstacles in our life. Sometimes you might see his body with the head of a falcon. This is not animal worship. We are admiring the attributes of the falcon and are striving to become that. Our ancestors personified the animal's strengths and survival techniques through science.

What do we know about falcons? They are one of the fastest predators. They devote themselves to one partner for their reproductive years (a lot of you guys can learn from the falcon). Heru's right eye represents the sun's ability to see all things. The bird is analytical and strategic. Horus or Heru is your willpower, transformation, vision, and control. Falcons signify attentiveness.

If you are too close to a sticky situation, you must step all the way back and rise above it. Now that you are high in the sky, having a bird's eye view of the situation, your perception and focus is increased, and now you can make a conscious decision. Our ancestors meticulously studied nature for thousands of years in order to create a system for their nation. There are hundreds of anthropomorphic representations you can research yourself. I just wanted to give an example of one in particular whose "logo" is seen worldwide.

Unlike major worldly religions, in ancient African spirituality God was not male. NTR was both male and female divine. You can find this clearly represented with the original and first "cross," which is an Ankh. The circle part of the Ankh represents the woman's womb and the straight piece below represents the male penis. It is the Symbol of Eternal Life. The divine was not created or centered around a male figurehead; there was balance throughout.

Kings and Queens (Pharaohs) were personifications of God on earth. We deified ourselves. We all have the capacity to be Buddha or Jesus. Under the Pharaoh's rule, you were not told how to think. You were encouraged to question everything and experience what was taught for yourself. There was no blind faith. Like I said earlier, heaven and hell are within you. The devil is the person or thing in your life creating your hell. That person can even be you.

Our early ancestors were mostly vegetarian, especially the priestesses and priests. Their diet consisted primarily of fruits, vegetables, beans, lentils, kamut, spelt, barley, and a host of herbs used for seasoning and healing. This is our original diet, people. There is no group of people who becomes powerful without investing in their history. Returning back to spirituality, clean foods, and right thinking right here in America will have our people investing in themselves and each other once again. To learn more about the African contribution to the world you can check out this amazing easy to read book, *Nile Valley Contributions to Civilization* by Anthony T. Browder.

COLONIZER OCCUPANCY

Black people ruled northern Africa up until 525 B.C. There were families that ruled for a considerable number of years. These families built the pyramids, libraries, and temples. The African people were architects, engineers, artists, designers, scientists, doctors, priests, etc. They were nowhere near an uncivilized race. An uncivilized race invaded their land, destroyed/stole their artifacts, imitated and brought some with them back to Europe.

From 3100 (the first Dynasty) to 657 (25th Dynasty) Africans ruled Northern Egypt, with the exception of 1750-1552 B.C. when the land was invaded by the Hyksos (a barbaric race). You can research this information. I won't go into a lengthy lesson about that invasion. Here are the major foreign successive invasions that ruined Kemet listed by year and invader:

- 525-405 B.C.E (Before common era) -PERSIAN RULE

- 404-343 B.C.E -NATIVE REVOLT (EGYPT RULED BY EGYPTIANS)

- 343-332 B.C.E -SECOND PERSIAN RULE

- 332-30 B.C.E -GREEK PERIOD (Alexander the Greek made all Kemetic spirituality illegal)

- 30-395 A.C.E -ROMAN RULE

- 395-640 A.C.E -BYZANTINE PERIOD

- 640-PRESENT DAY- ARAB RULE (This is why the face of present-day Egypt looks how you see it now. They are not the original inhabitants)

If you still don't believe ancient Egyptians were black, here are facts from an ancient European. The so-called "father of history," Herodotus said, "It is certain that the natives of this country are black with the heat..." and, "My own conjectures were founded, first, on the fact that they are black skinned with woolly hair."

---

71. Walker, Robin. *The Rise and Fall of Black Wall Street and the Seven Key Empowerment Principles*. Reklalw Education Limited, (2016), Pg. 14

72. Joshua Bloom and Waldo E. Martin, Jr. *Black against Empire. The history and politics of the Black Panther Party*. Oakland, California (2016), pg. 43.

73. Joshua Bloom and Waldo E. Martin, Jr. *Black against Empire. The history and politics of the Black Panther Party*. Oakland, California (2016), pg. 75.

74. Joshua Bloom and Waldo E. Martin, Jr. *Black against Empire. The history and politics of the Black Panther Party*, Oakland, California (2016) pg. 188.

75. Joshua Bloom and Waldo E. Martin, Jr. *Black against Empire. The history and politics of the Black Panther Party.* Oakland, California (2016) pg. 189.

76. Diop, Cheikh Anta. *The African Origin of Civilization, Myth or Reality.* Presence Africaine, Paris, (1955), pg. 1

PART III:
STRESS FREE

19

FIGHT OR FLIGHT

Fight or Flight (FOF) is a physiological reaction in the body that happens when a life-threatening situation arises. FOF is in the sympathetic nervous system (SNS) and keeps everything in balance. The response is triggered by the release of hormones that prepare your body to either stay and deal with the threat or run away to safety. Muata Ashby describes the response like this:

"In a true crisis where there is imminent danger, the increased heart rate allows for blood to be pumped rapidly to the muscles, so they can be mobilized to run or fight, and to the lungs so the blood can be oxygenated to supply fuel to the muscles. Other physiological changes include dilation of the pupils, to give a larger scope of vision so one can better see their options of escape, increased blood pressure resulting from the increased heart rate coupled with a decrease in the diameter of the vessels (constriction), the mobilization of energy by releasing fats and glucose into the bloodstream, and a release of blood coagulation factors so that in the event of injury, the blood can clot quickly to minimize blood loss."[77]

When I read this, I thought it was so amazing that the body does that without any assistance from us. The unfortunate part of this FOF response is that many men of color are tapping into this feature in their body all the time. Whether it's getting pulled over by cops, fear of going to prison, confrontation with another male ego, trouble at work, or maybe even problems at home. This in-depth process takes a toll on the body if triggered when unnecessary.

Staying in flight or fight drains and weakens your immune system throughout the course of your life. Your body will continue thinking you're getting chased by lions in the Safari, when really someone stepped on your foot in the club and you're ready to rip their head off.

"The stress hormone creates lesions (tiny, microscopic scars) in the heart muscle which over a period of time can predispose to heart disease. The transient increases in blood pressure eventually cause the mechanisms involved in regulating blood pressure to malfunction, leading to permanent increase in the blood pressure, predisposing to a variety of diseases including stroke."[78]

What if you really are in imminent danger, the physical aspect of your body also rolls into effect. Your psoas muscle (the only muscle connecting your upper and lower half) activates to bring your body into a ball/fetal position to protect your vital organs from trauma. When that important muscle is not functioning, your body's natural response is now in danger of being delayed. The lion chasing you is about to have you for lunch. Why wouldn't that psoas muscle be functioning? Excess sitting! Sitting too much shortens the muscle, leading to tension in the hips, knees and backs due to other muscles trying to compensate.

This is one of the many reasons we need yoga along with meditation. See how this is all tying in? Although India is known for yoga, it is well documented and inscribed in the temples that our ancestors practiced yoga, also known in ancient Kemet as Smai Tawi. Something as simple as stopping and taking a deep breath from deep within the belly can calm an overactive mind.

A great natural herb remedy for stress is Ashwagandha. This herb increases thyroid production of T3 and T4 hormones, which calms and energizes the mind and body, regulates your heart rate and body temperature. This herb is known to decrease stress levels by 44% and cortisol levels by 28%. The thyroid gland (located in front of your neck) also regulates how fast your intestines process food with the release of the hormones into your bloodstream.

Quick note: Soy products contain a compound that inhibit thyroid function. If enough hormones aren't produced by this gland or are overproduced, you will experience weight loss or the inability to gain weight.

Melanin is part of your nerve transmission between the cells. It is in your adrenal glands which secrete adrenaline that gets your heart pumping. We will all experience stress, but the problem is staying in that state for long periods of time. The adrenaline gives you a quick boost of energy, but over time it is taxing on your system and leads to hypertension. If your body is in a healthy state and your organs are working efficiently, your body won't have to depend on adrenaline to give you that boost of energy which stresses the heart. You will have a steady and even flow of energy provided from your liver when crisis arises.

As mentioned earlier, stress reduces the digestive enzymes produced by our body naturally that are needed to break down food. When you are in crisis, your body knows you don't need food. You must already have the nutrients (from natural foods) readily available in your body when the stress comes. Artificial foods are busy robbing your body of nutrients, leaving you defenseless, which sends your blood pressure through the roof.

We have to change how we think and changing our diet can greatly assist with that, because having clean nutritious foods have a calming effect on the mind and have you prepared for the pressures of life. We have been led to believe we should never get angry or we shouldn't have strong emotions, and I completely disagree. The higher being has given us this tool because we need it in this world. The key is to not overuse and abuse this tool because over time, it will make you sick. It is okay to get upset. That is a natural feeling, but staying in that feeling for an extended amount of time makes it a mood and that mood creates toxicity.

77, 78. Ashby, Muata. *Kemetic Diet; Ancient African Wisdom For Health of Mind, Body, and Spirit. Based on the Natural Diet and Health System of Ancient Kamit and Nubia.* Second Edition, (2002), pg. 116.

20

CHILL OUT

STOP

Some people only have true peace of mind when they are asleep. The purpose of this section is to begin to unlock your hidden potential and find ways to gain freedom from stress and mental imbalance. Two people can have the same exact issue and one person is stressed, but the other is not. It's all in how each person perceives that issue that can lead to stress or understanding.

An essential part of managing stress is learning to STOP. We shouldn't react to a person or situation immediately, while allowing our emotions to rule us. One of the most difficult things I have found in my journey is mastering the art of STOPPING. I'm used to reacting to a situation immediately, dwelling in my thoughts, feeding the pain, while getting carried away into the ocean of misery. Our ancestors practiced yoga and meditation to help them with "mind control."

WHAT IS A THOUGHT?

I came across an interesting lecture by Dr. Jewel Pookrum about mind and body connection. She describes the chemical reaction to thoughts in your body as this: Your brain translates all thoughts and reduces them to a vibratory rate so they become physical. The physical manifestation of a thought is known as a neurotransmitter. A neurotransmitter is a chemical released into the bloodstream and through every nerve in your body so that every cell knows what you are thinking. See the sketch below to understand what is happening.

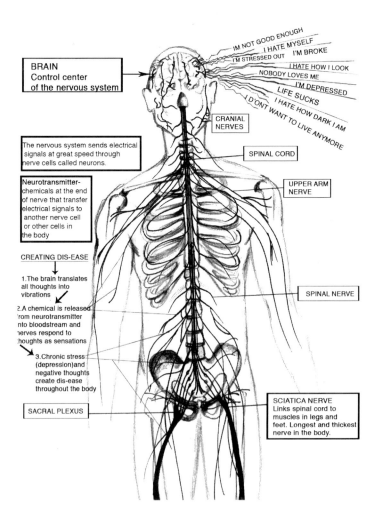

Your body then gives you the response to that thought by the sensations you have. So when you have thoughts that are toxic to the cells, that chemistry then causes the cells to react in such a way that provokes and gives you the feedback sensation of pain and discomfort. I found this information so interesting and it makes so much sense to equate mental stress to the physical stress of the body. Dr. Pookrum also mentions that our society has a tendency to run to the pharmacy and start popping Advil, Tylenol, and Motrin.

What these pills do is numb the nerves so that they cannot respond to the chemistry in your blood stream. None of these pills erase the chemistry that is going on from the stress trigger in your body. Melanin stores memory.[79]

Re-align your thoughts so that the chemistry shifts in your blood stream. High blood pressure, diabetes, heart disease, Alzheimer's, and every chronic disease is due to a chronic state of consciousness as well as diet. "Your cells will then respond and let you know that you made the shift, because you will have spontaneous healing from the tissues correcting themselves."[80]

WATER, SLEEP & DEEP BREATHING

Water is necessary to sustain proper function of the brain. It is essential to life, not just a casual drink to have when you feel like it. If you drink more liquor than water, you are on a fast road to weakening health. Water washes away those chemicals formed from negative thoughts that Dr. Pookrum mentions, so they can filter out of your body.

The brain contains about 75% water, and dehydration can alter its function. Anti-depressants impact serotonin (the happy molecule) which is naturally occurring in our body when we have diet high in natural foods. Based on people that I know, I've noticed that anti-depressants have an interesting way of keeping you depressed, especially when you're not hydrated. Instead of being stuck in that mentality of suffer-ing, water can help shift your consciousness. That is amazing! Drinking purified water - typically spring or distilled water, helps improve circu-lation, increases energy levels, and mental and physical coordination. Tap water is toxic. More than 60,000 chemicals are used within the United States.

Tap water is filled with chlorine, aluminums, lead, and nitrates. These toxic metals are a leading cause of brain damage and slow devel-opment in children, and kidney damage. Your kidneys' job is to filter and clean the blood by removing toxic chemicals and turning them to urine.

These toxic metals have a negative effect on your pineal gland which produces that important melanin we discussed in Part 1. They cause what's called a calcified pineal gland. As fluoride accumulates in the pineal gland, it hardens due to crystal production, which causes a lot of issues. One of many being melatonin and serotonin hormone reduction. Too much fluoride can throw off your circadian rhythms (twenty four hour clock.)

Studies have shown that patients with Alzheimer's disease have a high level of calcification in their pineal gland. Melatonin is responsible for fighting those free radicals that damage our bodies and speed up the aging process. The pineal gland is very sensitive to chemicals.

In general, you want to drink half of your body weight in ounces. I am usually around 150 pounds, so I would drink 75 ounces of water a day. If buying bottled water is too annoying, invest in a water filter and change it monthly or however often the manufacturer recommends you change it. Don't just keep the same filter for five months because you'll be breeding bacteria to put right back into your body. The goal is to decalcify your pineal gland and nourish those melanated centers in your brain.

Sisters and brothers we need to start getting more rest. Your body needs rest in order to repair tissues, rejuvenate, and heal itself. It is your body's way to ward off infection or dis-ease. Ongoing sleep deprivation is linked to heart and kidney disease, high blood pressure, diabetes and stroke. When we sleep our bodies rest- conserving energy while decreasing heart rate, blood pressure and body temperature. Focus and reaction time will be improved with adequate amounts of rest.

You will notice with an adequate amount of rest, your brain will function at optimal levels. You need to give the cell phones a rest and sleep in complete darkness, as that will also help activate your pineal gland to produce melatonin for healing. As soon as you wake up, drink one glass of room temperature water to activate your organs. Cold water is taxing on the body because now it has to do additional work to bring it to normal body temperature. Seven to eight hours of sleep per night is recommended.

Deep breathing has so many benefits. It cleanses the blood, calms an over-thinking mind, and improves oxygen and nutrient transport, while strengthening the lungs. We can manage a few days without water, but only seconds without oxygen.

Good breathing is essential to relaxation, easing tension, and promoting calmness. Under stress we tend to breathe short or hold our breath in. You have to remember to take a deep breath when faced with alarming situations. Most men are "chest breathers," meaning that breathing from deep in the belly and from the diaphragm (filling the lungs completely) is unusual for you. But that's where the calming/cleansing breath is formed.

Belly breathing maximizes oxygen intake and releases more toxins. A few times a day, just close your eyes and breathe in through the nose for five seconds out of the nose for five seconds. Belly breathing may not be comfortable for you at first, but it is extremely beneficial. Try to equalize your breath. Some of us inhale longer than the exhale or vice-versa. Breathe in-2-3-4-5 as your belly expands, and out-2-3-4-5 as your belly contracts bringing your navel to your spine. This should help relax and release any tension in your body.

The deep breather enjoys more peace of mind. If you practice deep breathing, you will think more clearly and sharply because you are stimulating your brain cells. Deep breathing in nature is excellent, because you're around less contaminated air compared to the city. So take a deep breath, fill up those lungs and that stomach, and allow your brain to relax.

MEDITATION OVER MEDICATION

So many of us are walking around with emotional baggage/wounds from our childhood and don't even know it. We picked up behaviors from our parents that were either positive or negative to our overall well-being. We go from relationship to relationship with negative habits that are our road blocks to healing. We question our self-worth and go into a depressive state.

I know for a majority of us it is completely unintentional. For me, intention is extremely important. Some of us have had great childhoods and some a complete nightmare. It's time to release the blame and take responsibility for becoming the person we want to be. Blame keeps you as the childhood person you want to escape. Responsibility is the rebirth of yourself and a chance to start over.

We don't have a choice when we are kids and learn from watching. That is over now and it's time to move on. These habits or cycles of

negative behavior can be reversed with the practice of mindful meditation. Don't be afraid to set boundaries and take time for yourself to
do the work to get you on the road to a positive mental well-being. If
psychotherapy is not an option for you, please consider energy therapy.

The mind is so wild and being a human is filled with so many
ups and downs. If we can train our minds to be more open and accept-
ing toward all experiences, whether good or bad, we can become more
relaxed, no matter what life throws at us.

**Meditation is a way of contacting the inner energy that pow-
ers the process of self-realization and self-healing**. There is a mystical
component of meditation that just cannot be explained, only felt. This
deep state of "being" is enhanced with a stimulated pineal gland. From
my experience, nourishing your pineal gland will give you access to different energies not available to just anybody. The feeling is unexplain-
able and almost unimaginable until it happens to you. It's the vibrations
or frequencies that lets you appear to be out of your body looking down
at it. People of African descent have been conditioned to believe that
our ancestral practices that deal with elevating the level of consciousness are evil. You have been taught this because you have special powers
that aren't available to just anybody.

You will learn how to train your mind, which changes your brain,
and experience the present moment. It is learning to work your mind
through whatever is going on. This allows your brain to determine
the difference between real danger and you just being emotional over
something. Meditation keeps you out of the fight of flight response.

The Buddha said, "The only thing I teach is suffering and the ces-
sation of suffering." Pleasure and pain are inevitable. We aren't trying
to run away or avoid the painful or stressful parts of life. I'm not saying you will no longer feel grief, pressure, physical pain, or negative

emotions. Rather, we want to have an awareness of what is going on in the present moment. In sitting meditation, thoughts will come and go like waves in the ocean. Meditation allows you to be receptive to whatever life brings you and to let go. We're not trying to stop the thoughts because resistance will make the thoughts stronger. Watch them come and watch them go.

There are many forms of meditation but the one I find most beneficial is where you just allow yourself to be. You sit down with your eyes closed (also can be done with eyes open) and allow yourself to experience what is going on, without judgement. This is not a competition for "who can have a blank mind the longest."

When a thought comes, acknowledge it, and say "bye" when it is ready to leave. Meditation can be done anywhere from five minutes to five hours. If five million thoughts come about, then accept what is happening without judgement. Spending time alone is not the same as feeling lonely. This is the prescription required for growth.

As you meditate, you will understand yourself more. We can locate those habits and patterns that are limiting our life. We think we know ourselves until we sit there and clearly see the thoughts that pop up in our head. I learned a lot about myself and when I started meditating. I realized how crazy I am. Just kidding, but I definitely learned how to control my thoughts better and truly live in the moment.

There's no such thing as meditating wrong. It's a gradual process. The goal is to not react based on habitual emotions or impulses within your control. Make a conscious decision as your mind is newly focused.

My insight to write this book came from meditating on the beach in Guanacaste, Costa Rica. Due to all the distractions in life, and giving my love and attention to everyone more than myself, I was missing out on my purpose in life. During sitting meditation on the beach, while decalcifying my pineal gland in the sun, it hit me! Then when I got back home from vacation, I realized I had been writing the book for almost ten years without realizing it. I started typing right away and the words flowed on the paper like water. When I started taking twenty to thirty minutes a day to meditate to take time just for me, it was so peaceful, even with the constant chatter in my mind.

Meditation allows us to break down how we have been conditioned and stop punishing ourselves over and over again with our thoughts. You will find that there is no need to react to every single moment. You also won't hold on to the feelings which can create disease. You will truly become flexible and at peace. Always ask yourself, "Is this something outside of my control that's happening or is it in my mind?" Being flexible and not reacting to every moment is key. It takes approximately eight weeks straight of meditation before your brain starts changing, so stick with it.

MINDFULNESS

Although unknown by many, our ancient African ancestors practiced meditation to achieve a high level of spirituality. A simple practice of mindfulness is a great way to start us on our journey to freedom from over-thinking, which usually leads to stress. Mindfulness is to be in the moment. Mindfulness means pay attention. Don't think about yesterday or tomorrow; just be right here.

Instead of allowing your mind to wander while performing any task throughout the day, just try to think only about what you are doing at the moment. If you are washing your car, do that – only think about washing your car. Chances are you will do a better job of it. Don't wash your car while thinking about the rent, mortgage, children's tuition, a break-up or anything that will take you away from being right here and right now.

When we ruminate on the past, we self-torture, which causes more pain to ourselves than any outside source can. When you think about a break-up, you relive that moment over and over again, bringing up all that negative emotion. There is no reason to lose yourself in the past or future, especially when your mental well-being affects your physical well-being. We punish ourselves one thousand times more than anyone else can because of our thoughts.

When you find yourself in a stressful situation, as difficult as it may seem, find conditions in your life that you can still be happy about. We all suffer to some extent and that's expected. Acknowledge what's causing the pain, look deeply into it to see what brought it about and stop ingesting thoughts to add to that pain. Once you do that, you'll see that you're already on the road to liberation.

Think about when you have back pain, a toothache, or any type of ailment that immediately puts you in misery. That is usually the only time you appreciate not having those ailments, but once they're gone, you go back to not appreciating good health anymore. We must be grateful every day and eat to preserve health and the well-being of our mind, body and spirit.

Don't ignore your pain because resistance makes the pain stronger. You can't fool your body – believe me I've tried. Acknowledge and look deep into it while still enjoying the positive aspects in your life right now. Looking deep into its meaning. Is it physical pain? Physiological or psychological? Buddhists believe, "without suffering, you cannot grow." I believe that myself.

In ancient Kemet, our ancestors aspired to overcome their lower-self to attain mental well-being and the highest level of spirituality. Your lower-self is your weaknesses, uncontrollable sexual appetite, eating immoderately, cheating, lying, stealing, etc. It is referred to as "Set" in Kemetic spirituality.

What is now called our present day "hell," in ancient times was a state of mind. Hell was not a place; it was a battle between your strengths and your weaknesses (state of mind.) This "hell" can be a good thing, as it challenges us and can lead us to growth and transformation. That's why in ancient Kemetic myths, the purpose was never to eliminate your lower-self (Set) because there would be times where you would need to be that person. You just allowed it to remain dormant until it was time to come out.

It's natural for your mind to drift in daily activities, but just come back to the present moment. Negativity affects the mind and the mind affects the body. We need to be aware of our thought patterns, habitual thinking, and belief systems, as these too can be culprits that trigger stress.

Our focus needs to be to get rid of the stressor and create some type of plan to re-train our brain and body on how we will respond to the experience the next time. It is imperative that we have new responses to reoccurring situations to prevent the release of the toxins in our bodies from the neurotransmitters in our brain. **Change your response, change your chemistry, and begin healing.**

You were not given the ability to think in order to inflict pain on yourself over and over again. I believe the reason for the amazing and mysterious ability to think is so you can attract what you want and communicate with a higher spirit. We underestimate the fact that we are our thoughts and our thoughts can control our destiny with a positive mindset. See what you want in detail, focus on it, and watch what the universe does for you.

Our ancestors did not focus on habitual negative thinking. They focused on right thinking; that is still attainable for us. Their heightened level of thinking allowed them to build the great pyramids and temples. We are the oldest recorded civilization on earth. That counts for a lot.

Dr. Pookrum said something important during her lecture on, "The Differences between Africans and other races and cell regeneration." She said, "The Universe rearranges itself to create your reality."[81] I find this to be so powerful and true! Most people don't get what they want because of their addiction to negative thinking which draws negative results to them. Work on not allowing your thoughts to take you away from the present moment!

Mindfulness can be practiced while you are:

- Eating (be mindful of chewing and experiencing all the flavors in your mouth)

- Walking (pay attention to your surroundings)

- Driving (Do not text, go on social media, or day dream – just pay attention)

- Give yoga a try. Being mindful of your body, postures, and your breath.

PERCEPTION & ATTACHMENT

Attachment to things and people causes a great deal of stress. The stress tackles us full force because we want things to be permanent that are not. Knowing this, we need to cherish the people we love while they are here, knowing that one day, they won't be. Appreciating the quality of impermanence will allow us to treat and speak to people in a decent manner.

Some of us have a very harsh way of speaking to our friends, man/ woman or people in general. You think it's okay because you're being honest. What you're doing is causing someone else pain or suffering. We may not realize this, but people treat you how they treat themselves and feel about themselves. Quite frequently people are treating you based on this story that you created in your head of how you think they're treating you. This is why we need to be mindful.

Mindfulness allows us to not let our perception create our reality. Our reality creates our reality. Take time to think about the person you're speaking to before you say something that can be damaging or hurtful. None of us want to experience pointless and avoidable suffering.

Let's work on being more understanding towards the people we love because love is understanding; and understanding doesn't mean agreement. It means having compassion. Before you speak ask yourself this:

- Is it true?

- Is it necessary?

- Is it hurtful?

- Is there a way I can phrase this to not sound hurtful?

Once we have a mind, body, and soul connection, we are unstoppable! Meditate to learn your mind. Once you learn your mind, work on slowing down useless thoughts. Those useless destructive thoughts create a chemical imbalance in our body causing nutritional deficiencies. In a chronic depressive state, those thoughts will lead to disease.

We all need to find our purpose. Some of us have not activated our souls and are not truly living. We must get our nutrition in order to balance out our body which will strengthen our minds. I have researched about whether the gut can heal the brain or does the brain heal the gut. I am on the fence and believe it can go either way. I believe even if your mental state isn't right but you change your diet, naturally, you will have a more positive mindset.

I changed my nutrition first because I was sick and tired of being sick and tired. I was able to conquer my illness and ailments. The mental growth came in years later, but physically I felt great. For those who believe they have a mental disorder, first things first – stop believing it. Second, you need to get your nutrition in order to balance out all the chemical reactions in your body from food and medication. The food is affecting your brain!

In reverse, I do believe a positive mindset can heal diseases as well. The mind is the most powerful force in the world. Negative thinking connected to past experiences is creating a toxic internal environment. If you stay in the moment you won't associate every thought with a feeling.

Remember, psychology tells us that the brain doesn't know the difference between an imagined experience and a live one. What you visualize is your brain's reality. Those who have purpose and a strong support system are usually very strong mentally and can heal themselves of every situation that crosses their path.

Purpose is so important, so if you don't know yours, try meditating; silence the world and find out. Once you find your purpose, visualize that purpose every day with a well thought out plan and watch your life begin to change. Science cannot answer all the questions about the mysteries of this world, only you can. If only we could get on the path to activating that force and aligning with nature.

Our ancient ancestors were more in touch with nature and the environment. They were nowhere near as contaminated as we are today. Access to a particular kind of energy was available to them because they nurtured their melanin.

Through meditation and clean eating, I was able to get a taste of that particular energy that is almost unheard of today. It is absolutely life changing when you experience it. Today we are drowning in another culture's way of living which is artificial and damaging to our lives. Melanin protects us and once you realize that, it will start working for you the same way it did for the ancients.

Meditation Key Takeaways:

- Decide what time you will practice meditation.

- Pick a consistent location where you won't be bothered.

- Burn some sage or incense to calm your nerves.

- Have a comfy pillow to sit on (or chair if you have back pain).

- Start with five minutes and increase to thirty minutes.

- Rest your hands on your thighs, palms down in a comfortable place that won't cause your back to round.

- Close your eyes
  (some people practice with their eyes open).

- You may feel restless, like you can't relax. This is completely normal.

- Place attention on your breath. If you feel your mind is too active, try counting your breaths. Ex: breathe in for four seconds, allowing your chest and stomach to expand. Pause at the top for a second and breathe out completely for four seconds until your stomach sucks all the way in. 1-2-3-4-pause-4-3-2-1-pause (repeat).

- When your mind takes you somewhere else, come back to your breath. You can also try eight seconds. Ex: Inhale for 1-2-3-4-5-6-7-8-Pause for four seconds - Exhale completely for 8-7-6-5-4-3-2-1.

- When the mind wanders and inner chatter begins, return to the breath to stay focused.

- Do not try to push away the thoughts, acknowledge them without judgment and slowly return back to the breath. Breathe in deeply filling up the lungs and stomach, and breathe out slowly releasing all negative energy and discomfort.

- There is no good or bad; only if you were mindful or not.

- Get to know the quality of your thoughts. Is your mind calm or busy? Is it a turtle or a race horse?

- Be sure to have a strong posture so the energy can flow from the bottom of your sacrum (tail bone) to the top of your head (crown). Remove all tension from your body.

- If your back starts to curve, straighten up. (Be aware)

- Try meditating in nature as it has a calming effect.

- NEVER GO TO SLEEP WITHOUT MEDITATING (PRAYING) ABOUT WHAT YOU WANT TO HAPPEN IN YOUR LIFE.

Mindfulness Key Takeaways:

- Mindfulness decreases depression, stress, tension, and anxiety. It boosts the immune system, improves memory, and increases focus/attention span.

- A positive mindset shift is one of the most important things we can do if we are going to overcome chronic pain and stress.

- Forgive yourself for anything dwelling in your subconscious mind.

- Our mind can be our source of suffering or our source of happiness.

- Remember, your mindset can give you a kick start forward in life, but it can also be what holds you back or sends you in reverse.

- Nothing changes unless something changes.

79, 80, 81. Dr. Jewel Pookrum. Published March 24, 2016. Differences between Africans and other races and cell regeneration. https://youtu.be/yJIF6BYS9po

FINAL THOUGHTS

There's an interesting process that happens to a divine being when he/she begins to understand the laws of nature and when he/she begins to understand themselves. There's a great transformation of your old self withering away while the new you emerges like a sunrise. There's a particular process in nature I have never been able to grasp, or understand, but it absolutely fascinates me. I want to share that with you before we close.

Metamorphosis is a biological process of transformation typically referenced when speaking about animals or insects transitioning from an immature form to an adult form through cell growth and differentiation. I want to break down the wondrous process of change from a caterpillar into a butterfly. It is one of the most stunning sights that is barely even thought about. The process is known as Chrysalis.

The butterfly starts life as a wingless caterpillar that develops in an egg. The caterpillar chews its way out of the shell and starts feeding on the leaf. The insect spends several days eating and growing plumper and longer while shedding its skin. After about thirteen days, the caterpillar hangs upside down from a twig, goes on a fast, and stops eating. A few hours after shedding its skin, it begins to reveal this beautiful, bright green skin called chrysalis, similar to a cocoon.

Eventually the old skin falls off and the bright green chrysalis is the only thing attached to the twig as the transformation begins. The caterpillar begins to digest itself, releasing fluids caused by hormones to dissolve all of its tissues. Nature programmed each cell to self-destruct to begin the metamorphosis. There are these cells called "imaginal discs" that survive the digestive process. Before it hatches, it grows an imaginal disc to fuel the cell division required for each of the body parts it will need to morph into a butterfly. These imaginal cells naturally kick into action once the caterpillar is wrapped in the chrysalis. Where did these imaginal discs even come from? Nature is amazing!

The caterpillar's cells completely disintegrate; imaginal cells create the wings, antennae, legs, eyes and all the features necessary for the butterfly's body. The imaginal disc can begin with fifty in the beginning of the process and end with 60,000 by the end. The butterfly emerges as the chrysalis splits open. It then pumps fluid from its body into the veins of the wings to expand and then flies away. Can we give nature a round of applause, please?

Metamorphosis is not just a beautiful physical transformation, it is a fascinating display of how two different species can emerge from one body. Butterflies and caterpillars LOOK NOTHING ALIKE. Really think about this for a second. They don't behave the same or even eat the same.

This story is relevant to the topics in this book because we are trying to kill our old, destructive selves. We want to self-digest the poisons that have been fed to us mentally, physically, and spiritually. The caterpillar stuffed his face until he couldn't take it anymore. The ignorant black person drinks and eats himself into oblivion due to stress and lack of knowledge of self.

Self-digest everything negative about yourself. Digest any form of self-hate that exists within your mind. Digest the history you have been taught in school that told you, you came from nothing. Digest anyone who told you, "you aint shit." Lastly, self-digest all the poisons from the unnatural foods, smoking, and drinking; and watch it eliminate from your body.

Become the butterfly and watch how your life morphs towards greatness. Remember, the people that created the problems cannot be part of the solution. You can do it!

"Every day, we have an opportunity to create the life we want."

ABOUT
SHANEEQUEWA SAMUELS

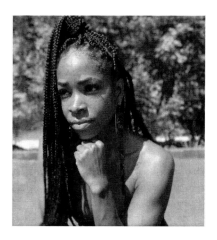

In 2009, Shaneequewa Samuels adopted a lifestyle of fasting, raw vegan diets, and clean eating, after having several inconclusive blood test results during 2008. She was disconnected from everything she would need to bring her body back into balance. She had left her religion for personal reasons, leaving her "spiritless." She ate a diet high in fast foods, animal protein, white processed foods, excess sugar, and no foods found in nature leaving her "nutrition-less." Lastly there was no physical fitness in her life at all, leading to the breakdown of her physical body.

She was in and out of the hospital for eight months and experienced fevers, vomiting, weakness, and severe joint pain at the age of twenty-six. She knew things were getting bad when she was barely able to walk due to severe pain in the knee joints. The final straw was when she blacked out, hit the floor, and lost her vision for just a few minutes. This was her final time in the hospital where she was told again that they didn't see anything wrong with her they could label with a brand name dis-ease. She concluded she wasn't sick enough for them to diagnose her.

She was determined to find a balance between her soul, mind, and body. This traumatic experience led to the reversal of dis-ease in her body and revitalized her as a person. She adopted a raw vegan diet along with a full body cleanse in 2009 where she went from 145 pounds to 129 pounds in a matter of three months. This allowed her to overcome all her ailments that Western medicine wasn't able to treat. This experience was the driving force behind her ultimate change.

Shaneequewa also began a strict workout regimen where she learned the essentials of functional movement. Her first major experience with training came from pole dancing and CrossFit. These two activities built the foundation for what would ultimately become her lifestyle. Within the ten years of learning about the body's capability of healing itself, she spent eight years studying African Spirituality and Meditation, which greatly allowed her to truly get to know and love herself. After overcoming numerous ailments, her transformation and journey led her to become a Certified Holistic Nutritional Counselor and share her experiences and knowledge to help others heal themselves.

ACKNOWLEDGMENTS

I want to show love specifically to the men of color who have been a true inspiration in my life whether it was directly or indirectly. They've been there for me through pivotal events in my life, some life changing. Regardless of how society decides to portray men of color, they are amazing fathers, brothers, protectors, and creators.

Vincent "Uncle Vern" Roper, Safaree "Scaff" Samuels, Cursy "Kreyol Flavors" St. Surin, Kevon Samuels, Jamain Adams, Justin Adams, Robert "Rubskin" Garcon, Keon "Keez" Watson, Raymond Muscat, Robert Clark, Vladimir Destinoble, Darren "Dwat" Watson, Glentis Dye-Michel, Devon Mitchell, Kareem Baptiste, Reggie Gray, Marc "Marvelous" Innis, Howard "Ho-Ho Cakes" Grant, Prince Goulbourne, Paul "Pandemonium" Jean-Louis, Peter Brooks, Amir Wilson, Jorde Adams, Brandon "Byrde" Brown, Saiquon "Sai" Kirkland, James "Supa" Britt, Omar "Sugar bear" Simmons, Raul Arroyo, Lionel Canton, and Michael Jeffrey.

Your encouragement, assistance, and companionship often sustained me during the preparation of this work, and for that, I THANK YOU!

RECOMMENDED READINGS

Readings to Free your African Mind:

1. *Stolen Legacy – The Egyptian Origins of Western Philosophy* by: George G.M. James

2. *They Came before Columbus – The African Presence in Ancient America* by: Ivan Van Sertima

3. *Christopher Columbus and the Afrikan Holocaust-Slavery and the Rise of European Capitalism* by: John Henrik Clarke

4. *Precolonial Black Africa* by Cheikh Anta Diop (He was an Egyptologist, Nuclear Physicist, linguist, and Politician)

5. *The Autobiography of Malcolm X as told to Alex Haley*

6. *African Origins of the Major Western Religions - The Black Man's Religion Volume 1* by: Yosef A. A. ben-jochannan

7. *Black Man of the Nile and his Family* by: Dr. Yosef A.A. ben-jochannan

8. *Post Traumatic Slave Syndrome- America's Legacy of Enduring Injury and Healing* by: Joy Degruy, Ph.D

9. *The Isis Papers - The Keys to the Colors* by: Dr. Frances Cress Welsing

10. *African Holistic Health* by: Llaila O. Afrika